KU-539-478

LEEDS BECKETT UNIVERSITY
LIBRARY
71 0198199 TELEPEN
DISCARDED

ENDOCRINOLOGY

MANAGEMENT OF COMMON DISEASES IN FAMILY PRACTICE

□ □ □ □ □ □ □ □ □ □ □ □

Series Editors: J. Fry and M. Lancaster-Smith

ENDOCRINOLOGY

□ □ □ □ □ □ □ □ □ □ □ □

P. Marsden, BSc, MD, FRCP

Consultant Physician,
Greenwich District Hospital

and

A. G. McCullagh, BA, MB, BCh

General Practitioner, Lakeside Health Centre,
Thamesmead

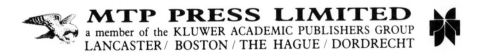

MTP PRESS LIMITED

a member of the KLUWER ACADEMIC PUBLISHERS GROUP

LANCASTER / BOSTON / THE HAGUE / DORDRECHT

LEEDS POLYTECHNIC
478151
DISCARDED
78
18.6.86
616.4

Published in the UK and Europe by
MTP Press Limited
Falcon House
Lancaster, England

British Library Cataloguing in Publication Data

Marsden, Philip, *1941–*
    Endocrinology. – (Management of common diseases
    in family practice)
    1. Endocrine glands   2. Diseases
    I. Title   II. McCullagh, A.G.   III. Series
    616.4   RC648

    ISBN 0-85200-865-1
    ISBN 0-85200-794-9 set

Copyright © 1985 P. Marsden and A. G. McCullagh

All rights reserved. No part of this publication may be reproduced, stored in a retrieval system, or transmitted in any form or by any means, electronic, mechanical, photocopying, recording or otherwise, without prior permission from the publishers.

Typeset and Printed by UPS Blackburn, 76-78 Northgate, Blackburn, Lancashire.

Contents

□ □ □ □ □ □ □ □ □ □ □ □

Series Editors' Foreword

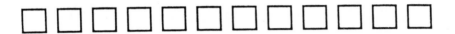

Effective management logically follows accurate diagnosis. Such logic often is difficult to apply in practice. Absolute diagnostic accuracy may not be possible, particularly in the field of primary care, when management has to be on analysis of symptoms and on knowledge of the individual patient and family.

This series follows that on *Problems in Practice* which was concerned more with diagnosis in the widest sense and this series deals more definitively with general care and specific treatment of symptoms and diseases.

Good management must include knowledge of the nature, course and outcome of the conditions, as well as prominent clinical features and assessment and investigations, but the emphasis is on what to do best for the patient.

Family medical practitioners have particular difficulties and advantages in their work. Because they often work in professional isolation in the community and deal with relatively small numbers of near-normal patients their experience with the more serious and more rare conditions is restricted. They find it difficult to remain up-to-date with medical advances and even more difficult to decide on the suitability and application of new and relatively untried methods compared with those that are 'old' and well proven.

Their advantages are that because of long-term continuous care for their patients they have come to know them and their families well and are able to become familiar with the more common and less serious diseases of their communities.

This series aims to correct these disadvantages by providing practical information and advice on the less common, potentially serious conditions, but at the same time to take note of the special features of general medical practice.

To achieve these objectives, the *titles* are intentionally those of accepted body systems and population groups.

The *co-authors* are a specialist and a family practitioner so that each can supplement and complement the other.

The *experience bases* are those of the district general hospital and family practice. It is here that the day-to-day problems arise.

The *advice and presentation* are practical and have come from many years of conjoint experience of family and hospital practice.

The *series* is intended for family practitioners – the young and the less than young. All should benefit and profit from comparing the views of the authors with their own. Many will coincide, some will be accepted as new, useful and worthy of application and others may not be acceptable, but nevertheless will stimulate thought and enquiry.

Since medical care in the community and in hospitals involves teamwork, this series also should be of relevance to nurses and others involved in personal and family care.

JOHN FRY
M. LANCASTER-SMITH

1

INTRODUCTION

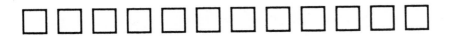

NATURE OF ENDOCRINE DISEASE

Endocrinology has something of a reputation for abstruseness among general practitioners. The diseases are often thought of in a general way as being rare and of only peripheral interest to the average family doctor. This viewpoint has of course some basis in relation to some endocrine conditions but it is far from the truth. Endocrine conditions affect all age groups and vary greatly in their prevalence from diabetes mellitus and thyroid disease, where we can expect one sufferer in the average roomful of people, to very rare conditions such as testicular feminization. A Royal College of General Practitioners' survey showed that the average general practitioner is likely to see seven thyroid cases and ten new diabetics every year. On the other hand he or she may never see a case of Addison's disease. Many endocrine diseases have a reputation for rarity when they are in fact quite common. Hyperparathyroidism (occurring in around one per 1000 of the population) and Klinefelter's syndrome (affecting about one in 600 live male births) are two examples. The second major point of interest about endocrine disease is that it is, by and large, eminently treatable and treatment can usually restore a normal or near normal lifestyle.

Although there are many causes for endocrine dysfunction and the pathological basis for disorders of the endocrine glands is

1

varied, the clinical manifestations tend to be grouped around the hormonal effects of the glandular secretions – that is, they reflect the absence or lack of hormone or its effects when present in excess. Hormones of course act on cells and we now recognize the importance of the cellular receptor side of this relationship in causing endocrine dysfunction. Many conditions, including common ones such as obesity and some types of diabetes and rare ones such as pseudo-hypoparathyroidism and testicular feminization, can now be looked at in a new light as disorders where the hormones may be present and correct but there is a defect in cellular responsiveness.

Endocrine diseases, then, can be looked at in one way as disorders of communication between cells and, because hormones such as insulin, thyroid hormone and cortisol act on not just one target organ or tissue but on a great variety of tissues, the effects of endocrine dysfunction and the corresponding clinical features of endocrine disease are often 'cellular' or multisystematic rather than locatable within an organ/system structure for classifying disease. It is because so many non-endocrine disorders can be classified in this way, and we so often think along these lines when presented with a clinical problem, that endocrine disease can be missed. Thus the sufferer from myxoedema with watering eyes is often sent to the ophthalmologist, with aching limbs to the rheumatologist, with carpal tunnel syndrome to the orthopaedic surgeon, with constipation to the gastroenterologist, with falling hair to the dermatologist and finally with thyroid function tests to the endocrinologist.

One of the purposes of this book is not just to add to the doctor's knowledge of endocrinology but to change that knowledge qualitatively so that it becomes more useful and accessible in the recognition and management of people with disorders of the endocrine glands.

SPECIAL PROBLEMS

It is true unfortunately that endocrine disease often presents late and is subsequently not ideally managed and followed up. There are of course other reasons for this in addition to the one given above concerning the internal organization or structure of the doctor's knowledge about endocrine diseases and its attunement to the clinical presentation of these disorders. One of the foremost of these is, firstly, that endocrine disorders are usually of slow and insidious onset before diagnosis and, secondly, that they run a chronic course after diagnosis.

There are relatively few acute syndromes in endocrinology but those that do occur can be extremely dangerous and need always to be in the forefront of our minds. Hypoadrenal crisis, diabetic ketoacidosis and hypoglycaemic coma, visual compression from a pituitary tumour and pituitary apoplexy, post-thyroidectomy (or parathyroidectomy) hypocalcaemia, thyrotoxic crisis and malignant exophthalmos are some of the most important. In general, these and other endocrine disorders tend to progress slowly and all too often with 'non-specific' symptoms such as 'tiredness', emotional and mood change and a sense of poor bodily function that are all too readily categorized as functional.

Another reason for late recognition is that diagnosis is so often laboratory dependent and in the past the inaccessibility and complexity of many of the tests used to assess endocrine disorders has inhibited the involvement of the general practitioner. Often these procedures have meant hospitalization or have only been available in large teaching centres with many resources and staff. This situation is now changing rapidly. The past 20 years have seen an enormous increase in our ability to measure hormones in blood largely through the advent of ever more sensitive and specific radio-immunoassay techniques. At the same time tests have simplified and often require no more than a venous sample of blood to measure a specific hormone present in a concentration that even 10 years ago would have seemed unthinkable. Simplification of techniques and the advent of systems like the supraregional immunoassay service have meant that many of the essential investigations are within the reach of general practitioners with local hospital agreement. It is time for the mystery surrounding endocrinological tests to be shed and a new era of understanding and involvement for the general practitioner to begin.

ROLES OF GP AND CONSULTANT

As indicated above, a further aspect of endocrine disease is the fact that many of the conditions are lifelong and their management poses particular problems in relation to monitoring and prolonged and effective aftercare. There is a very important role here for the general practitioner, since follow-up in specialized hospital clinics may require people to travel long distances, have time off work, and so on.

The general practitioner can help improve the standard of health provision for those with endocrine disease in yet another way. Many types of endocrine disease, in particular pituitary disease and gonadal endocrinology, require the services of more than one hospital-based specialty. For instance a person with a pituitary tumour will need to be assessed by the neurosurgeon and possibly the neurologist, the ophthalmologist, the neuroradiologist and the endocrine physician. He may also require the radiotherapist's help. Disorders of the gonads, including infertility, need expert help from the gynaecologist as well as the physician and the role of the chemical pathologist should not be forgotten. Very often the coordination of these services becomes extremely difficult in the long term and is in fact one of the major logistic problems in the management of endocrine disease. The general practitioner all too often plays a merely passive role whereas one suspects he or she should have a major role in ensuring continuity of care and screening and monitoring services.

The question of the most effective and economical way to deliver complex health care to the community raises itself most particularly in areas such as thyroid disease and above all diabetes. The very high prevalence of diabetes in the community effectively ensures that the provision of effective diabetic care solely via the means of a hospital-based diabetic clinic is not practicable. While inside the hospital different systems for the provision of diabetic care (such as diabetic day centres, open access ward facilities etc) are being explored, the involvement of the general practitioners in primary diabetic care is becoming daily more important.

One of the problems in this situation is that, from traditionally

4

being asked not to be involved in diabetic care, many general practitioners have become extremely reluctant (and in some cases not able) to be involved. This is primarily a question of education and again of changing the knowledge we have so that it becomes more useful in practice. Probably some system of shared care involving effective mechanisms to ensure the appropriate screening and monitoring for each particular disease is the best way forward for the care of people suffering from chronic diseases of the endocrine system. Such a system must of necessity involve other members of 'the team' as well as the general practitioner and hospital-based consultant.

This book is intended to help the general practitioner in the recognition, assessment and long term management of those with endocrine disorders. Each chapter considers a particular endocrine gland and the content is organized so as to provide some basic factual information on the common diseases affecting that gland, the common presentations of disorders in terms of clinical manifestations and assessment and management. We shall try throughout to place the emphasis on clinical relevance and day to day management and to present the information in such a way as to allow the practising general practitioner to identify more easily those persons within his or her practice who are suffering from endocrine disorders to facilitate their assessment whether in the practice or at the hospital and to ensure their proper long term management.

The general features of endocrine disease, and endocrine emergencies, are summarized in Table 1 (overleaf).

Table 1   Endocrine disease: general features and endocrine emergencies

General features of endocrine disease
Very common and very rare clinical features varied – 'cellular' – not 'systematic'
Insidious onset – often missed
Chronic course – requiring long term monitoring

Diagnosis in many cases much simpler nowadays

Education 'block' to be overcome by GPs

Very treatable on the whole

Endocrine emergencies
Adrenal crisis
Diabetic ketoacidosis
Hypoglycaemic coma
Visual compression from pituitary tumour
Pituitary apoplexy
Hypocalcaemia
Thyrotoxic crisis
Malignant exophthalmos

2

THE PANCREAS

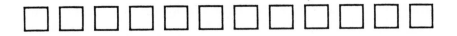

DIABETES MELLITUS – WHAT IS IT?

Diabetes mellitus is a disorder of carbohydrate metabolism resulting from a true lack or insufficient action of circulating insulin which results in hyperglycaemia. The condition arises from malfunction of the β-cells in the islets of the pancreas, or a defect in the action of insulin. We recognize two main types of diabetes:

(1)   insulin dependent diabetes (IDD), Type I diabetes,

(2)   non-insulin dependent diabetes (NIDD), Type II diabetes.

Most Type I diabetics are young people but unusually this type of diabetes occurs in the maturity onset years. Similarly there is a group of non-insulin dependent diabetics who present in youth (MODY – maturity onset diabetes of youth). This has an autosomal dominant mode of inheritance.

PREVALENCE OF DIABETES

Diabetes is a common disease present in about 1–2% of the population. Of these, about two thirds will have NIDD. Non-insulin dependent diabetes occurs most commonly in the 50–70 age group. Childhood diabetes peaks at 5 years of age and again between 10 and 12 years but is still uncommon, with a prevalence of 0.1%.

AETIOLOGY

Diabetes is a syndrome arbitrarily defined and the aetiology is not fully understood. There is a familial link in diabetes of both types. Genetic factors in diabetes are probably multiple and in most cases not very obvious in the individual case, except in rare syndromes and monozygotic twins with NIDD. It is important to realize that only 1% of children with one diabetic parent, and 5% of children with both parents diabetic, are themselves diabetic. The mode of inheritance has not yet been established in most cases. However IDD – but not NIDD – is associated with HLA antigens. Probably the effect of the HLA-associated genes is permissive, allowing the effect of, for instance, viruses such as Coxsackie B4 and mumps. Variations in the incidence of these genes may account for epidemiological difference in the prevalence of IDD. HLA-DR is also associated with other endocrine diseases such as thyroid and adrenal insufficiency and pernicious anaemia, perhaps providing the basis for the increased incidence of thyroid disease, pernicious anaemia and Addison's disease in insulin dependent diabetics. Another immune mechanism probably involved in the aetiology of IDD is the presence of pancreatic islet cell antibodies in some people associated with HLA antigens. It is postulated that genetic susceptibility to viral infection and subsequent auto-immune distruction of β-cells is the immune basis for IDD. The hypothesis of viral infection as part of the causative mechanism derives support from the seasonal incidence of IDD with peaks in winter and spring. There are also peaks in incidence at the ages of 5 and 11, perhaps related to school entry. Obesity is found more often in NIDD, where it may be related to the aetiology. Obesity is often associated with high serum insulin levels and insulin insensitivity. There are however, probably other factors operative in the causation of NIDD. Diabetes may also be associated with a number of other conditions such as acromegaly, Cushing's syndrome (includes exogenous steroid use) and phaeochromocytoma – conditions where an excess of insulin antagonists is present. In addition pancreatic disease, postpancreatectomy, pancreatitis or haemochromatosis cause diabetes, and drug induced diabetes occurs with injudicious use of corticosteroids, as mentioned, and with thiazide diuretics, the oral contraceptive pill and diazoxide.

DIAGNOSIS OF DIABETES

The diagnosis and definition of diabetes laid down by the World Health Organization is:

(1)   a fasting plasma glucose of greater than 8 mmol/l and/or
(2)   a 2 hour plasma glucose level of 11 mmol/l or more.

Impaired glucose tolerance

This is defined as existing when the fasting plasma glucose is less than 8 mmol/l and a 2 hour plasma level is between 8 and 11 mmol/l. A random level below 8 mmol/l or a fasting level below 6 mmol/l excludes both diabetes and impaired glucose tolerance. When glycosuria is found blood sugar should always be monitored, as glycosuria can occur in renal glycosuria which is a harmless condition. Note that in most diabetics presenting with glycosuria a simple random blood sugar will make the diagnosis. Thus a large group practice with 11 000 patients could expect to have about 100 – 150 diabetics on their lists if every case were detected and under treatment. The fact that many people suffering from diabetes live undetected for considerable periods is one of the major challenges to diabetic care. In many instances however even diagnosed diabetics do not receive ideal care. Diabetes is a common and easily diagnosed disease. Its treatment is eminently manageable by the general practitioner with other members of the primary health care team. Many of the current problems in diabetic care could be solved by better organisation of diabetic care and better education. The importance of patient education and motivation in such provisions cannot be overemphasized, but also of importance is the education of doctors and other health care professionals in diabetes.

THE PROVISION OF DIABETIC CARE

What problems?

Historically, the management of diabetes in Britain has tended to be under the control of the hospital outpatient diabetic clinic and the general practitioner seems to have been frightened of coping with his diabetic patients. This is largely the result of a level of education in diabetes for the majority of doctors at undergraduate and postgraduate levels which is not appropriate to the prevalence of the disease. This state of affairs is unfortunate because diabetes, once contracted, is a lifelong condition and the surveillance by the general practitioner under properly organized conditions is therefore not only appropriate but can make a very valuable contribution to welfare of individuals both medically and psychologically. Such a pattern of care also provides considerable benefit to the general practitioner in terms of producing good clinical records based on accurate and regular follow-up. It is now being recognized that the medical ('diabetic') outpatient clinics cannot themselves provide adequately for all diabetic care in a health district, and the pattern of care in diabetes is changing. One of the main changes afoot is based on the encouragement of general practitioners to manage the majority of their diabetic population themselves, with the consultant diabetologist and specialists of other disciplines providing back-up to deal with problems and complications as they arise.

The requisites for successful general practitioner monitoring of diabetes in group practice should probably be as follows.

(1) A special miniclinic run by the same doctor at regular intervals, i.e. once a fortnight.

(2)   The concomitant use of a practice nurse trained in diabetic care who will not only help in running the clinic but would also be able to do home visits to deal with queries on the spot and give appropriate advice or change in treatment.

(3)   The use of a diabetic recording card set separately from the normal notes, while patients also carry their own recording cards so that liaison between hospital and general practitioner where necessary is made easier.

(4)   Access to the diabetologist and hospital diabetic services.

(5)   Access to a diabetic dietician preferably on the same day as the clinic.

(6)   Access to an ophthalmology clinic.

(7)   An efficient recall system.

Our diabetic clinic cards are two-sided, as shown in Figure 1.

On the first side a general history and assessment both past and present is recorded and clinic attendance dates noted, and only any change in treatment recorded. On the reverse side the parameters are clearly indicated in histogram form. It is relatively easy to see how an individual is controlled. Spot random blood checks in the clinic may be inaccurate in assessing general control and the regular use of the glycosylated haemoglobin (HbAic) has been found to be a helpful indicator, giving as it does an index of average control over several weeks. It appears to correlate very well with clinical suspicion of poor control and to confirm when control is thought to be adequate.

The advantage to the patient of attending the practice clinic is that of ease of access and continuity with the same doctor. It is possible that more delicate problems such as impotence are more likely to be tackled than in the more impersonal hospital environment.

It is not only by provision of better diabetic care within the individual GP practice that changes are being instituted. The hospital-based diabetologist is also committed to changing the

ENDOCRINOLOGY

NAME	ADDRESS	DATE OF BIRTH	
CURRENT HISTORY	PAST HISTORY		
FAMILY HISTORY			
INITIAL ASSESS	SMOKING		

DATE	NOTES	TREATMENT	DATE	NOTES	TREATMENT

Figure 1 Two-sided diabetic clinic cards (front)

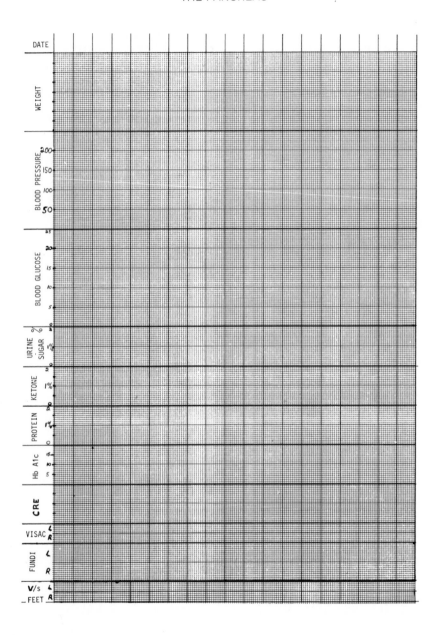

Figure 1 (back)

pattern of care and facilities for the diabetic person. Different health districts will to some extent have different needs and constraints, but in Greenwich the following summarizes recent developments and ideas:

(1)   The diabetic clinic. This cannot possibly cope adequately with the total provision of diabetic care and education. It continues to provide a vital interim role while the developments referred to below become available and effective. There will also be an important residual role.

(2)   GP education programme. As stated above, some GP practices are already heavily involved in diabetic care but others are not. There has been a reluctance amongst general practitioners to embark on diabetic care and, while there are other reasons for this, one of the most important reasons is lack of confidence due to lack of education. To encourage general practitioners we have set up a GP education programme including

    (a)   provision of experience in diabetes in hospital on a paid clinical assistantship basis,
    (b)   setting up of a joint hospital/GP diabetic club and
    (c)   provision of feedback educational pamphlets to GPs based on referral problems. One of these is given as an example (Figure 2).

(3)   The shared care scheme. For some time we have encouraged the setting up of GP miniclinics (largely for NIDD at first) with the following shared care provision:

    (a)   Use of a shared care booklet.
    (b)   Provision of yearly screening of visual acuity, fundus, feet, blood pressure, weight, urine, blood glucose and HbAic by the hospital clinic until the GP wishes to do this himself or herself.
    (c)   The idea is to encourage a circular movement of diabetics so that care is primarily in the community but access to hospital care is available urgently when problems arise. Both diabetic and GP are circulated with

Figure 2 Management of intercurrent illness in diabetes – suggested regime for primary care 2

When a diabetic becomes ill with an infection etc, the most important thing is the type of diabetes. Insulin dependent diabetes (IDD) needs much more careful handling, though non-insulin dependent diabetes (NIDD) must also be watched. One of the commonest causes of admission to hospital with diabetic ketoacidosis is the mismanagement of a person with IDD who has developed an intercurrent illness. Here are the Do's and Dont's.

IDD

Never ever stop insulin injections
A commonly reported story is that the patient stopped insulin because she was not eating. There is an endogenous requirement for insulin which is generally *increased* in an intercurrent illness.

So how much insulin does your patient need?
Look at the tests (urine and blood) and you will see. Whenever an illness strikes, the IDD patient must start testing four times daily if not already doing so. If the tests are uniformly high she or he needs *more* insulin, not less. If the tests are largely OK the insulin dose is also correct. Only if the patient is suffering hypoglycaemic reactions should the dose be decreased and this is very unlikely. It is helpful to also test for ketones four times daily, but not essential.

How do you increase the insulin, then?
While the tests are all high, advise that insulin be increased by 4 units *per injection* until 50% of tests are controlled. As the patient improves, reduce accordingly. If the patient is on mixed insulins increase the soluble component. If on a once daily injection, it sometimes helps to introduce a small evening dose of soluble 4 u at a time though often this is not necessary. This advice is given routinely to IDD patients attending my clinic.

What about food? — the patient may say he or she is not eating at all
It is essential that the patient keeps up carbohydrate intake according to the portions in his or her diet. So firstly, what is the diet? If the patient cannot take solid food then advise semisolid food or liquids or high glucose fluids.

Remember 10 g of carbohydrate (one portion) is contained in 6 fluid oz. (9 cl) of milk, 2 fluid oz. (6 cl of Lucozade, ½ fluid oz. (15 ml) of neat Ribena. Anyone who cannot keep down about ⅓ pint (about 20 cl) of Lucozade three times a day should probably be in hospital.

What are the danger signals?
If diabetic symptoms of thirst, polyuria and weight loss appear – transfer to hospital.

If ketones appear in low concentration intermittently without diabetic symptoms it may just be that enough carbohydrate is not being given. Heavy ketones or ketones with diabetic symptoms indicate the need for urgent transfer to hospital.

If you are out of your depth, transfer to hospital – then join the diabetic club.

(*continued overleaf*)

NIDD

In non-insulin dependent diabetes the risk of diabetic ketoacidosis is very small. The rules for testing and food intake still apply and also encourage fluids. In general sulphonylurea tablets can be increased by one tablet per day at 48 hour intervals up to the permitted maximum while tests remain high and reduced according to the same rule as things improve. It is permissible to allow some deterioration in control in such patients since they very rarely need insulin. Danger signals are as before – severe diabetic symptoms plus or minus ketonuria despite increasing the tablets.

---

pamphlets on the expected provision of care when first hospital follow-up ceases. One is given as an example (Figure 3). It will be noted that access to hospital care is available urgently for control problems, visual deterioration or foot lesions in addition to any referral on more general grounds or yearly screening appointments.

(4) The diabetic day care centre. The concept of a centre available on a day care basis for diabetics is now becoming accepted as providing the basis for better diabetic care. Not only can urgent problems be dealt with more efficiently but the opportunity exists for extended education and group work.

Several districts now have such centres already working efficiently, but where it is not possible to establish such a centre, or as an interim arrangement, it is possible to use (for instance) the ward as an open access area or other convenient site within (or outside) the hospital for provision of education programmes or group work (*see below*, on education of the patient).

Other developments in the provision of diabetic care are as follows.

(1) More widespread use of nursing staff in the education and management of diabetics. Development of clinics run by trained nursing staff and the encouragement of practice

You have now been discharged from the diabetic clinic but this does not mean that your diabetes is cured or that you should stop your diet, treatment or testing. Neither does it mean that we have forgotten about you. What it does mean is that we consider that you understand enough about your diabetes to be able to be more independent of the hospital, which is a good thing.

We have established a system of shared care in Greenwich for diabetics which means that from now on you will be looked after by your own doctor and the clinic.

Here are the rules and regulations:

(1) See your doctor three times a year
(2) *Continue* urine or blood testing, your diet and any tablets
(3) Record your results in the co-operation booklet with which you have been provided and take this with you to the doctor
(4) Every year you should be screened. This involves recording your weight, blood pressure, urine test for sugar and protein, blood glucose and HbA concentrations. It also involves looking at your feet and into your eyes. This can be done by your own doctor or here at the clinic (by appointment). We will not continue to follow you thereafter in the clinic unless there is a reason
(5) Always see your doctor if you are unhappy about your diabetic control, if you notice poor vision or trouble with your feet

If at any time you have a problem with your diabetes, see your doctor and if he or she agrees we will see you again in the clinic for a while until things are sorted out once more.

If you have any questions ask them now. If problems occur to you later ask your doctor or ring the clinic.

Your doctor knows about these arrangements.

Figure 3 Patient information on diabetic clinic 'discharge'

nurses trained in diabetes and diabetic liaison sisters (or clinical nurse specialists) one of whose roles it is to cross the hospital/community barrier

(2) Development of self-help groups and joint doctor and patient led groups, such as parent groups and adolescent groups led by specially trained young diabetics.

CLINICAL FEATURES

Presentation of diabetes

Diabetes can present itself in many different ways. The following are examples of presentation during a 3 year period to a GP clinic in South London:

- (1) vaginal candidiasis refractory to normal treatment
- (2/3) myocardial infarction
- (4) leg ulcers
- (5) furunculosis
- (6) poor coordination (the patient noticed his darts playing had deteriorated before admitting to diabetic symptoms on closer questioning)
- (7) paraesthesiae of hands and feet
- (8) classical polyuria and polydipsia
- (9) balanitis
- (10) routine urine testing
- (11) referral from optician
- (12) weight loss

It is very important to note the distinction between IDD and NIDD in terms of clinical features.

In IDD:

- (1) the person is usually young
- (2) the onset is acute or subacute (and may be very acute)
- (3) diabetic symptoms are almost always present: thirst, polyuria and weight loss and a feeling of being unwell
- (4) ketones are present on testing the urine

In NIDD:

- (1) the person is usually of middle age or above
- (2) the onset is gradual
- (3) diabetic symptoms may be present but are often absent or dismissed
- (4) ketones are usually absent

For the GP assessing the urgency of an uncontrolled and perhaps previously undiagnosed diabetic, proceed as follows:

(1)   Is this or could this possibly be IDD? If so, then urgent referral is preferable unless you are confident.

(2)   Assess severity of lack of control by reference to the presence of persistent heavy glycosuria, diabetic symptoms (presence and degree) and ketones (presence and degree).

(3)   Blood sugar estimations are helpful but remember that blood sugar values of up to 25 mmol/l occur in NIDD, may have been present for some time and usually respond well to oral hypoglycaemics. Postprandial values may be alarmingly high even when there is only moderate loss of control in NIDD. The age of the patient, the degree and duration of symptoms and the presence of ketones are usually more reliable indicators than a single blood sugar estimation unless it is very high.

In NIDD the gradual onset means the condition is often missed (a good argument for routine urine testing) or, more tragically, diagnosed and then 'forgotten' about. The patient often presents with complications of diabetes such as visual loss or foot problems.

Screening for diabetes

Screening a whole practice population for diabetes is probably unrealistic and unrewarding. However, certain age groups with recurrent problems perhaps increase the index of suspicion and it may be that these individuals could be picked up by selective screening processes as the average time between onset of symptoms and diagnosis may be several years.

Morbidity of diabetes

Despite the advent of insulin therapy the prognosis for diabetics is not good and the morbidity remains high. This is of course largely due to the late complications of diabetes – microangiopathic disease in the retina and kidney, peripheral neuropathy and atheroma affecting the major blood vessels. In recent years, however, studies on retinal complications of diabetes do show that good diabetic control has a beneficial effect on retinopathy and of course the effects of excellent diabetic control in pregnancy have revolutionized the outlook in terms of fetal mortality. Although absolute proof is lacking it is the general consensus that it is appropriate to strive to attain normoglycaemia in diabetes in order to try to avoid the onset of microangiopathic complications. The development of atheroma in diabetics may be related to factors other than hyperglycaemia, such as raised plasma lipids. All diabetics should now be encouraged to follow a diet low in fat and high in vegetable fibre.

MANAGEMENT OF THE DIABETIC

What are the aims of treatment?

These are:

(1)   in all diabetics, the return to and maintenance of the ideal body weight for height and age and sex,

(2)   to control by the use of diet, exercise, oral hypoglycaemic agents or insulin the metabolic abnormalities of lipid and sugar, and

(3)   to attempt to prevent long term complications by means of the first two aims.

Education of the patient

Diabetes is a lifelong condition and it seems sensible that those who suffer from it should be given the greatest encouragement and opportunity to understand their condition and to control it. Patient education – or rather the education of those children, parents and adults who suffer from diabetes – is now assuming increasing importance in diabetic care. It is our responsibility not just to tell diabetics what they should know but also to tell them why, in terms and in language that they can relate to. This latter point is assuming greater importance because of a widespread feeling that nurses or perhaps even other diabetics may make better diabetic educators than do doctors. As doctors however we must be primarily concerned in consultation with other members of the team in defining what the diabetic should know and what overall tactics and strategies can be used to improve diabetic care.

One development stemming from educational theory has been the consideration of the 'behaviour gap'. In simple terms this means that you cannot assume that what has been taught has been learnt, and it is learning that is important, not teaching. Because of this many centres are now developing 'educational objectives' for diabetics which are stated in terms of what the diabetic person must be able to *do* to demonstrate that he or she has learnt. For instance, rather than have a check list of things the patient has been taught (itself an admirable thing when judged against the provision of no formal educational programme) we can now ask the patient to demonstrate that he can, for example, actually test his urine for sugar, or do a home blood glucose monitoring profile, or that as an IDD he does actually carry sugar on his person, now, this morning. A list of objectives for NIDD as used in Greenwich is shown in Figure 4.

Such developments allow us to begin to frame an educational programme for diabetics. This will differ for different types of diabetes or special groups such as adolescents or pregnant diabetics but basically the educational programme provides a tactic for fulfilling the aims of management by encouraging self-help and also the involvement of all members of the team rather than just the doctor. All diabetics in the UK should be encouraged to join the British Diabetic Association.

The non-insulin dependent diabetic should be able to:

(1) *Define* diabetes in terms satisfactory to the educator. Explain diabetic symptoms.

(2) *State* that treatment involves primarily diet and exercise and then tablets if necessary in addition. Never tablets alone.

(3) *State* that the aims of treatment are to lower the blood sugar to a safe level to avoid immediate symptoms and long term complications.

(4) *State* the effects on blood sugar of exercise, carbohydrate food and tablets.

(5) *State* that the 'sulphonylurea' tablet that they have been prescribed should be taken before food at times of day acceptable to the doctor and food must never be omitted after the tablet has been taken. If on metformin, state that it should be taken immediately after food.

(6) *Demonstrate* to the satisfaction of the educator urine testing with Clinitest or Diastix.

(7) *State* an acceptable frequency of testing.

(8) *Demonstrate* acceptable records of urine testing.

(9) *State* that hypoglycaemia is a blood sugar that is too low. State that it is caused by missing meals, taking too many 'sulphonylurea' tablets or excessive exercise only in those on 'sulphonylurea' tablets. State the symptoms satisfactorily.

(10) *Demonstrate* if taking sulphonlyureas that they carry sugar on them. State when to take.

(11) *State* that when ill they will (a) test at least three times daily (b) increase their tablets × 1.

(12) *State* that they will seek medical advice when (a) they are not confident what to do, (b) they do not improve, (c) diabetic symptoms appear, (d) urine tests do not improve.

(13) *State* that their diet is (a) reducing, (b) high fibre/low fat/sugar free.

(14) *Produce* written documentation of their diet.

(15) *State* that they will consult their doctor or optician immediately if they notice impaired vision.

(16) *Produce* a foot care document and describe their own procedures satisfactorily.

(17) *State* the requirements of the Driving and Vehicle Licensing Centre (DVLC) and insurance companies with regard to driving.

(18) *State* the need for continued supervision.

(19) *State* the need for yearly screening of blood sugar, blood pressure, eyes feet and weight.

(20) *State* the reasons for shared care. State their intentions to visit their doctor three times yearly routinely and be screened by GP or clinic yearly. State they understand their diabetes is not cured on discharge from the hospital clinic. State that they intend to continue diet, testing and tablets if prescribed.

(21) *State* that they know that smoking is dangerous and that they are advised to stop.

(22) *Produce* the home blood glucose monitoring documents and describe to the educator the advantages and uses of profiles and to document hypoglycaemia. Demonstrate procedure (optional).

Figure 4 Educational objectives for non-insulin dependent diabetics

MANAGING THE NEW NIDD DIABETIC

In the GP clinic

In Thamesmead I always attempt to explain what diabetes is in lay terms and stress the importance of diet, giving up smoking and assessing one's own control by means of regular routine urine and/or blood testing. Regular attendance at the clinic is under-lined, and any problems which may arise the community nurse or myself will be available to deal with by telephone or home visit. The dietitian will always see her own patients and arrange follow-up. Following the introduction the diabetic nurse carries out the routine parameters on the chart and instructs the individual in blood or urine testing. BM stix are useful adjuncts to be used at home. Unfortunately these are not yet available on F.P. 10 and so another source, usually a friendly hospital pharmacy, has to be found.

In the hospital clinic

For a newly diagnosed NIDD we would aim to control the diabetes (*see below*) appropriately while commencing the educational pro-gramme (*see* Figure 4). When the person completes the prog-ramme he or she is discharged to the shared care scheme as previously outlined. We will see the patient urgently as shown in Figure 3 – and yearly for screening purposes. Both the diabetic person and the general practitioner are given a written statement indicating the expected level of diabetic care for the future.

THE NEW INSULIN DEPENDENT DIABETIC

Probably most new IDD are still admitted to hospital in Britain today but there is a widespread move to try to avoid this. Certainly centres provided with a diabetic liaison sister are able to com-mence insulin administration directly in the clinic and follow-up the patient carefully at home. It is certainly helpful to prepare either check lists or, better still, behavioural educational objectives for IDD, in order to monitor and space out correctly in time the learning experiences which the new IDD needs to undergo. For instance probably the most vital thing is for the diabetic to inject him or herself with insulin *ab initio*. It is also vital that hypoglycaemia is understood and the necessity for carrying sugar to counteract it is understood and complied with. Other learning, such as home blood glucose monitoring, can come later. These observations apply to those IDD patients who feel well at presentation. Anyone who is unwell with serious metabolic derangement or drowsiness must be admitted to hospital. Provided the patient is sufficiently intelligent and motivated, there is no reason why a district nurse who has received special training in diabetes cannot instruct the patient at home in self-injection and administration of insulin.

DIET

Diet is the first line of treatment in all diabetics. All diabetics should receive dietary advice. Dietary recommendations for diabetics have changed markedly in recent years. Whereas formerly the emphasis was on carbohydrate reduction and intake of fat and protein was relatively controlled, modern diet favours a controlled fat intake (about 30% of total calories) and the use of unrefined carbohydrate rich in vegetable fibre to constitute 55 – 60% of total calories with about 60 g of protein per day. A lot of emphasis is placed on high fibre foods such as oat, wheat bran, sweet corn, kidneys, beans, broccoli, wholemeal bread and so on. Vegetable fibre slows glucose absorption from the gut and reduces peak glucose levels. Sugar and foods containing sugar should be avoided and foods containing sorbitol (diabetic preparations) have no indication for usage. The diet should be realistic for the patient – some F-plan diets can be expensive – and the energy content should maintain ideal weight and satisfy hunger. Therefore all obese diabetics should be on a reducing diet. If the person is not obese carbohydrate content can vary between 100 g and 300 g a day depending on energy expenditure. In the non-insulin dependent, 'foods freely allowed' and 'foods freely avoided' are useful guidelines. Those on sulphonylureas, however, should always phase meals with maximum time of action of the tablets, and those on long acting preparations must take a bedtime snack. In the insulin dependent diabetic the diet must also be more consistently arranged in terms of grams of carbohydrate exchanges according to the insulin regime. An exchange is 10 g of carbohydrate. Sensible advice on alcohol should also be given and at every possible opportunity the diabetic should be reminded to give up smoking. It is very important that diabetics have access to the skills of a dietitian. All GPs should be able to name the carbohydrate exchange value of common foods such as bread, milk, potatoes, fruit, cereals and beer and to make a rough calculation of the carbohydrate content of a diet.

Figure 5 illustrates the spread of IDDM and NIDD in a group practice of 11 000 with age of onset.

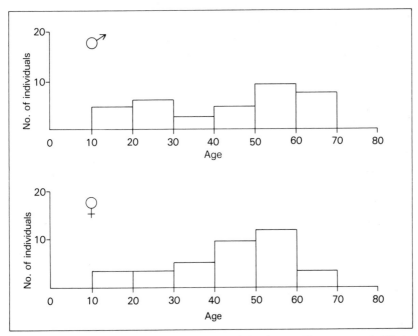

Figure 5 Age/sex distribution of new diabetics at Thamesmead Clinic (in decades)

INSULIN THERAPY

A working knowledge of the types of insulin available including their relative times of onset and length of action is mandatory. There are wall charts available from different drug firms and a monthly update in MIMS magazine to refer to (Figure 6). Nowadays there is no justification for the use of old-fashioned 'dirty' insulins in new patients or in any patient who has problems with insulin injection or diabetic control or who needs a large dose of insulin. Purified pork insulins are less antigenic than beef and human insulin should be considered particularly for use in children. This knowledge should be passed on to the patients so that they understand the mode of action of the insulin they are injecting themselves with.

Injection regimes

A typical regime may consist of one daily injection of a medium acting insulin, a daily injection of a short and medium acting insulin or a morning and evening injection of a medium and of a short acting insulin. Nowadays, and certainly in the younger patients, two injection regimes are encouraged. The aim of insulin therapy is to attempt to attain normoglycaemia throughout the 24 h period and to avoid hypoglycaemia especially during the night. Insulin dosages may have to be altered according to stress factors, lifestyle, whether it is the weekend or whether the individual is on shift work. All newly diagnosed IDD patients are now taught to self-adjust insulin dosage. Regular meals with a known carbohydrate content should be taken throughout the day. The actual types of food taken are varied, keeping the carbohydrate content the same by use of carbohydrate exchange values for different foods (10 g per unit). It is usual to inject 15 – 30 minutes before food. A typical intake of carbohydrate is 150 g split into three units of 40 g with three small snacks of 10 g in between meals to avoid hypoglycaemic attacks. A carbohydrate snack should always be taken before bed.

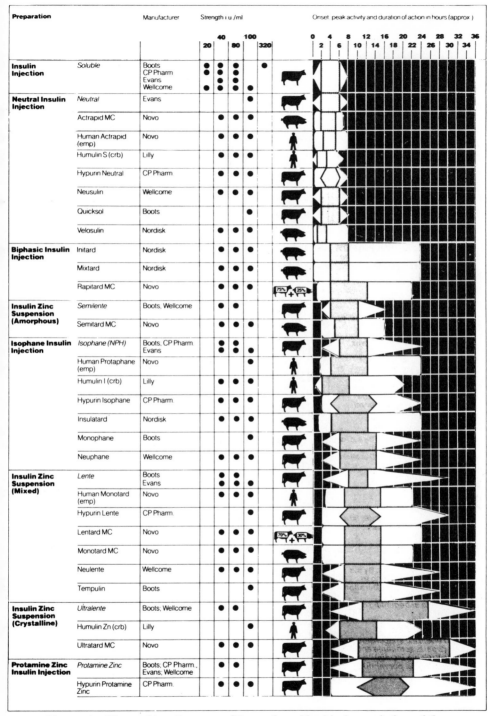

Figure 6 Chart of insulin types. (Reproduced by kind permission of the publishers of MIMS. Copies of this chart appear regularly each month in MIMS)

Monitoring

All patients should test their urine and/or their capillary blood for glucose at regular intervals and should adjust their insulin dosage on the results. There are advantages and disadvantages to both systems, but most IDD, particularly if young, are now encouraged to do home capillary blood glucose monitoring which allows much tighter control. Clinitest tablets are more accurate than Clinistix and are to be preferred for urine testing. They do however deteriorate in the light and in damp and if they change colour should be discarded and replaced. Diastix are both convenient and reliable. For home blood glucose monitoring a reflectance meter can be used or a strip test such as BM stix which does not require a meter.

Urine should be tested at the time of maximum activity of the insulins which the patient is taking so that the dose may be safely increased if sugar is found. In general, testing before the main meals of the day is found to be appropriate. Since with a normal renal threshold glucose does not appear in the urine until the blood glucose is 10 mmol/l, urine tests should in general be negative for sugar to indicate reasonable control.

Home blood glucose monitoring should be done as a profile of values about four to six times in 1 day on 2 days a week – unless the person is out of control, when more frequent testing is necessary.

Sick day rules

It is essential that all IDD patients understand what to do when they become unwell, are under stress or cannot eat. These are the rules:

(1) Never stop insulin.

(2) To know how much insulin you need – test. As soon as illness strikes, commence monitoring four times daily if not already doing so.

(3) If tests are high (urine or blood), increase insulin by

2–4 units per injection until at least half the tests are controlled (negative urine or blood glucose less than 10). Reduce similarly as the illness abates.

(4)   Test for ketones daily.

(5)   Watch for diabetic symptoms; thirst and polyuria.

(6)   If you cannot take solid food you must keep up your carbohydrate intake with high glucose fluids. One carbohydrate exchange (10 g) is contained in 2 fluid ounces (60 ml) of Lucozade, 1 tablespoon neat Ribena or 1 glass of milk.

(7)   If you are not confidently in control, call for help sooner rather than later.

PROBLEMS WITH INSULIN THERAPY

Pragmatic

Often when insulin therapy is started a 'honeymoon period' occurs, during which, owing to some recovery of β-cell function, the required dose of insulin drops for a few weeks or months. Insulin dosage must be reduced to prevent hypoglycaemic attacks. It is important that all those who start on insulin should be aware of the symptoms and causes of hypoglycaemia right from the start. All IDD patients should carry sugar on their person always. Anyone in Britain commencing insulin therapy must inform the Driving Vehicle Licensing Centre (DVLC, Swansea) and their insurance company if they are drivers. Instructions as to what to do if a hypoglycaemic attack occurs while driving should be given – stop, remove the ignition key, move into the passenger seat and take sugar.

Psychological

Psychological problems occur in some diabetics in association with insulin therapy largely to do with resentment that diabetes should affect them or reluctance to take insulin injections. Unfortunately certain age groups are less likely to be motivated than others. The adolescent male or female can be extremely difficult to motivate as diabetes tends to interfere with his or her lifestyle. These people need particular reassurance and encouragement. Adolescent girls particularly tend to deliberately overdose themselves or avoid taking their insulin often because of underlying emotional problems. When this kind of behaviour occurs management can be difficult, requiring interpersonal skills of a high order. Nowadays adolescent groups are being established so that the better-motivated adolescent can help those with problems. Sometimes hospital admission may be the only way of assessing whether insulin dosages are being taken in the correct and regular manner.

Biological

Acute allergic reactions can occur, particularly with insulins that have not been highly purified and with beef insulin. Local reactions that may occur at injection sites include fatty lumps and fat atrophy; the remedy is to avoid the sites and change to highly purified insulin. Review insulin injection techniques, which should involve rotation of injection sites. Occasionally infection, bruising or scars from intradermal injection occur at insulin injection sites.

New U-100 insulin

Since the early part of 1983 the United Kingdom has been gradually changing over to the new 100 u per ml concentration. This move means a gradual removal of 20, 40 and 80 strength insulins. This makes the administration of insulin theoretically more simple and less liable to produce mistakes. It brings Britain into line with Australasia, Canada, the United States and one Scandinavian country. Other members of the European Community and members of the communist block show no indication of changing at the present time – which means warnings should be given to patients who are going abroad.

THE NON-INSULIN DEPENDENT DIABETIC

Diet and exercise are the cornerstones of treatment. Encouragement is vital. If after several clinic attendances blood sugars are still raised and glycosuria is still present, then oral hypoglycaemics may be added provided diet has been encouraged. The sulphonylureas are usually the first choice. These act by stimulating insulin release from the β-cells of the islets in the pancreas. They also unfortunately stimulate the appetite and so it may become more difficult for the individual to lose weight. There are many different preparations on the market – one to avoid in the elderly or those with renal impairment is chlorpropamide since this has an extremely long half-life, is renally excreted and can produce profound hypoglycaemia as it accumulates over a period of weeks or months. Modern sulphonylureas include glibenclamide, glipizide, glibornuride and gliclazide. All sulphonylureas can cause hypoglycaemia. The second group of drugs are biguanides, now largely available in Britain only in the form of metformin. These can be used separately or as an adjunct. They act chiefly by reducing liver glucose production but also by impairing glucose absorption from the gut and increasing peripheral tissue glucose uptake. They do not stimulate insulin release and do not cause hypoglycaemia. Metformin is not as well tolerated as the sulphonylureas, causing anorexia, nausea, vomiting and diarrhoea and a general feeling of ill health. The biguanides also cause lactic acidosis. Phenformin is contraindicated and metformin should be used only with caution in the presence of hepatic, renal or cardiac failure. Alcohol consumption can also precipitate lactic acidosis in those on biguanides.

WHO NEEDS INSULIN?

Insulin dependency is the rule in the young, where there is often a rapid onset of symptoms with ketosis. Insulin dependency is in fact recognized by the presence of persistent hyperglycaemia, prominent symptoms and above all ketosis. Tablets are not given in pregnancy. If diet fails to control blood sugar levels then insulin is given. Poorly controlled, 'maturity onset' diabetics may need to be switched to insulin after some years. This so-called secondary failure occurs in about 10% of NIDD patients.

COMPLICATION OF DIABETES

Hypoglycaemia

The insulin dependent diabetic is at far greater risk from hypoglycaemia than is the diabetic on sulphonylureas. He or she should be aware of the symptoms and the action to take, including always to carry sugar on his or her person. Relatives should also be aware of how to deal with the situation.

Case report is an account of a wife describing her husband, an insulin diabetic for 15 years, normally stable, having a series of hypoglycaemic attacks in the early hours of the morning.

He had taken his normal insulin the evening before. The wife said:

> At 2.30 a.m. I woke up to find my husband thrashing about in bed. He sat up, and I noticed one side of his body was not moving. He couldn't speak, and was grunting loudly. He was dripping with sweat. I tried to get some sugar into him orally which was very difficult as he was violent and confused. He eventually took some and after $1\frac{1}{2}$ hours went to sleep. It was very frightening. In the morning he was quite all right except for a splitting headache. He remembered nothing of this. The same thing happened two nights later.

It transpired that he had not been eating properly because of worry over a sick relative. Dietary advice, stricter BM stix testing over a few nights and a minor adjustment of his evening insulin prevented any further problem of nocturnal hypoglycaemia. The wife was also instructed to administer glucagon intramuscularly if this should occur again.

She was in fact unable to administer glucose to him and has now been issued with and instructed how to use glucagon.

Diabetic ketoacidosis

Ketoacidosis with its concomitant hyperglycaemia, dehydration and electrolyte disturbance is an emergency and the patient should be admitted to hospital as soon as possible. Diagnosis is usually straightforward and can be confirmed on urine or blood testing. The detailed management will not be further considered here, but these are the principles:

(1) Replacement of fluid intravenously: use normal saline, 2 litres in 2 hours and then 1 litre every 3 hours;

(2) In the presence of marked acidosis administer sodium bicarbonate solution;

(3) Insulin is administered intravenously by infusion pump – 6 u per hour;

(4) Intravenous potassium replacement should commence with either bicarbonate or insulin administration.

For the GP the following are useful points:

(1) If the diagnosis is certain, administer 20 u of soluble insulin intramuscularly before transfer to hospital if this is likely to be delayed;

(2) Set up a saline infusion;

(3) Be aware of hyperosmolar (non-ketotic) diabetic coma.

A further role of the clinic is to assess and deal with complications as they arise.

The eyes

Visual acuity is recorded once a year when the pupils are dilated with a short acting mydriatic such as tropicamide 1% and the fundi examined. A deterioration in visual acuity of more than two lines on the Snellen's chart should always be double-checked by an ophthalmologist. We distinguish between background retinopathy consisting of microaneurysm, haemorrhage and hard or waxy exudate and the far more dangerous proliferative retinopathy where new vessels formed abnormally in an ischaemic retina can bleed, causing vitreous haemorrhage and blindness, or can lead on to fibrous retinitis proliferans which can detach the retina. The GP should therefore be familiar with the changes in the diabetic retina and learn to inspect the macula with particular care. In Greenwich, yearly screening is offered by the hospital for all patients of those GPs who are not yet able to examine the fundus with confidence. Maculopathy and proliferative changes can be detected early and are amenable to treatment with photocoagulation.

Microaneurysms are relatively harmless in themselves but indicate the need for heightened supervision. Exudates are important if they encroach on the macula. A ring of exudate around the macula may indicate maculopathy. Cataracts and glaucoma are seen in association with diabetic retinopathy. Nearly-blind diabetics should be encouraged to learn braille and join the talking book club.

Neuropathy

The commonest form of neuropathic complication is the peripheral neuropathy. This can be detected by the loss of vibration sense in the feet and absence of the tendon jerk. The symptoms are numbness, paraesthesia, or it may be symptomless. It can also be extremely painful. The pain of peripheral neuropathy is extremely difficult to treat and may require polytherapy in the form of tricyclic antidepressants and strong hypnotics. The health of the feet and toenails should always be checked and footwear reviewed for its suitability. Other somatic neuropathic complications of diabetes are isolated nerve lesions (e.g. oculomotor) and diabetic amyotrophy with painful wasted quadriceps.

Autonomic neuropathy

This may be concomitant with somatic neuropathy. It can produce various disturbances such as postural hypotension, tachycardia, gustatory sweating and in the male, impotence. Diarrhoea may also be troublesome. There are various methods for testing the presence of autonomic neuropathy – a simple procedure is to test the variation of the heart beat during deep breathing in the normal subject. There should be a variation of at least ten beats between maximum inspiration and maximum expiration. This variation is lost in autonomic neuropathy. Hypotension can be troublesome and in some cases can be helped by wearing full-length elastic stockings and by a high salt diet. Indocid is often helpful. Mineralocorticoids (fludrocortisone) can be given. Diarrhoea may be controlled by codeine phosphate.

Impotence

This is not uncommon in the diabetic and it is important to distinguish between functional and organic impotence. This first requires careful history-taking. Impotence due to organic disease tends to be slow in onset and permanent. There is loss of, or retrograde, ejaculation, decrease in libido and loss of early morning erections. Functional impotence tends to be of sudden onset and intermittent in its intensity. Morning erections are normally maintained. Tightening of diabetic control is indicated whether impotence is organic or psychogenic in origin and reassurance and encouragement should be emphasized. Mechanical aids should also be considered.

Nephropathy

Diabetic nephropathy is a longstanding complication and is of uniformly bad prognosis. Sixty per cent of diabetics are likely to develop nephropathy after 30 years and nephropathy is the commonest cause of death in diabetes. It is interesting to note that all nephropathic diabetics have retinopathy but not all retinopaths have nephropathy. The first simple mark of the nephropathic kidney is the presence of proteinuria in significant amounts. This may continue for many years and serum creatinine values will help to assess the problem more clearly. The rise of serum creatinine in a given patient can be predicted to indicate available time before renal support will be needed. Hypertension in association with renal failure should be vigorously controlled with the use of diuretics and selective β-adrenergic blockers. We now know that once significant proteinuria has been established, good diabetic control is unlikely to affect the outcome. However, it is hopeful that improved methods of detecting microproteinuria will allow detection of the disease at an earlier and reversible stage.

Diabetes in pregnancy

Optimum control of blood sugar is vital during pregnancy for the health of the mother but most particularly for the growing fetus which is seriously at risk if sustained hyperglycaemia is present, even when this is of mild degree. Pregnant diabetics should be under the close supervision of obstetric, diabetic and later paediatric specialists. In spite of great improvement in perinatal mortality in recent years in the diabetic due to improved control of diabetes, the mortality is still three times greater than normal, most of the deaths now being due to fetal abnormalities. The education of the pregnant mother really starts before conception as the fetus may be at risk of congenital abnormality if the diabetes is poorly controlled at the time of conception. So again motivation in the patient is of utmost importance.

SUMMARY OF DIABETES

Most diabetics can be managed for the most part within the context of the general practice, leaving the diabetologist more time for diabetic problems and the organization of educational programmes in diabetes for all concerned with diabetic care. Children, adolescents, the pregnant mother and complicated or problem diabetics are exceptions to the above statement and they should probably be managed at least initially by consultant care, and later perhaps on a shared care basis. There are at present attitudinal and educational constraints on general practitioners which limit their involvement in diabetic care but things are changing rapidly.

3

THYROID DISEASE

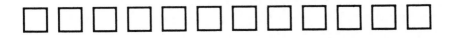

Thyroid disease will be considered under three headings:

Goitre

Hyperthyroidism

Hypothyroidism

GOITRE

What is it?

A goitre is an enlargement of the thyroid gland which may be either diffuse or nodular. Goitre occurs in association with both hyper- and hypothyroidism and when the patient is euthyroid. Goitres are extremely common (around 10% of the population in Britain). They affect women about ten times more often than men. There are major geographical variations in prevalence. The causes of enlargement of the thyroid gland are:

(1) *The action of TSH* on a gland which for varied reasons is unable to produce enough thyroid hormone:

    (a) autoimmune thyroiditis

    (b) congenital enzyme deficiencies in hormone synthesis (dyshormonogenesis)

    (c) drugs and dietary goitrogens

    (d) subacute (viral) thyroiditis

    (e) iodine deficiency

    (f) Riedel's thyroiditis

(2) *Neoplasm* – either primary or secondary,

(3) *Presence of abnormal thyroid stimulators* – TSH receptor binding antibodies in Graves's disease.

There are clearly many causes of goitre. Classical causes such as iodine deficiency are very rare in Britain, unless puberty and pregnancy goitres are considered as such. Dyshormonogenesis is also rare, unless nodular forms of goitre are considered as partial forms of this.

What problems?

The general problems are:

(1) *Identification* – many patients and their doctors are unaware that they have got a goitre. Partly this reflects the fact that the gland has not been examined or has been poorly examined but this fact must be considered also in relation to the significance of goitre.

(2) *Significance* – the majority of small goitres are of no significance and anxiety commonly ensues when these are identified *and then investigated inappropriately*. On the other hand pathological goitres tend to be under identified and therefore escape appropriate investigation.

Clinical features

Examination of the thyroid gland – general points

Both the general problems referred to above can be restated in terms of the clinical examination of the thyroid gland.

(1)   The thyroid gland is often missed out in routine examination.

(2)   It is often examined inadequately. The contribution of the condition of the gland itself to assessment of patients with hypo- and hyperthyroidism is large but it is often not mentioned in spontaneous accounts (referral letters; case discussions; presentations; reports; summaries).

This section therefore is designed to alter the way that doctors think about thyroid disease – *to emphasize the primary importance of the gland itself.*

When thyroid disease is suspected *first* examine the gland and *then* determine clinical thyroid status (Table 2).

Table 2   Assessment of thyroid enlargement *

Stage	Inspection	Palpation
0	Not visible	Not palpable
1	Not visible	Palpable but less than 40 grams (small)
2	Visible	Palpable but small
3	Visible	Palpable and more than 40 grams (large)

* Modified from Kilpatrick, R., Milne, J. S., Rushbrooke, M., Wilson, E. S. B. and Wilson, G. M. (1963). *Br. Med. J.*, 1, 29

40 grams is about a twofold enlargement of the normal gland. In the normal gland one can usually feel the isthmus but not the lobes

41

Clinical examination

(1) *Position* – don't stand behind the patient where you cannot see the gland. Usually a position to the side with one hand behind and one in front of the patient's neck allows both inspection and palpation. If necessary then go round to the other side to examine the lobe which is on your side of the patient; otherwise pronate the wrist of the hand examining the gland so that the thumb is down, which will also allow examination of the ipsilateral lobe.

(2) *Inspect* – during conversation with the patient when the gland is not being discussed. Swallowing movements often occur at this time. Otherwise a glass of water is an essential prop.

(3) *Palpate – anatomically:* both lobes; the isthmus; the pyramidal lobe.

(4) *Make particular note of:*

   (a) Consistency; firm and hard goitres may be Hashimoto's thyroiditis, neoplasm or Riedel's thyroiditis.

   (b) Nodularity; multinodular or a single lump. If a single lump, is the remainder of the gland impalpable (atrophied)?

   (c) Asymmetry; of particular importance – malignant goitres are often asymmetrical.

   (d) A bruit; only a systolic 'whoosh' over the gland alone, not venous hums, transmitted murmurs or large vessel bruits. Lymphadenopathy; it is most important when a goitre is thought to be pathological to examine for cervical lymphadenopathy, Horner's syndrome and recurrent laryngeal nerve involvement (hoarse voice). Any lump outside the position of the normal thyroid is suspicious though thyroglossal cyst should be borne in mind.

   (e) Size, Is the goitre very large? Is the trachea displaced? Is there retrosternal extension? Is there stridor?

Putting this all together

All this information is all very well, but what can we do to use the information more effectively? What general processes can be recommended for the doctor to assess goitre efficiently?

(1) Examine the thyroid gland routinely by inspection during conversation.

(2) When a goitre is noticed either routinely or as a result of medical enquiry:

    (a) *do not* tell the patient routinely or attribute neck symptoms to it expediently: *because* small insignificant goitres are the rule – thyroid neurosis is very common.

    (b) *do* examine carefully and make a judgement to refer (or manage appropriately) or reassure. GP follow-up without either specialized opinion or further investigation of suspect goitres is not advisable.

(3) Assess thyroid status after examination of the gland.

(4) The features that make a goitre suspect of malignancy are:

    (a) rapid increase in size – *this is the most important of all*

    (b) symptoms of pain, discomfort, breathlessness

    (c) extra thyroid swellings accompanying it

    (d) large size itself (stage 3)

    (e) lack of knowledge of a long stable history

    (f) firm or hard consistency

    (g) bruit

(5) Reassuring features are:

    (a) known long history without change

    (b) small size (stage 1 and 2)

    (c) symmetry   with no other suspect features present

    (d) soft consistency

Symptoms of goitre

Rather as in hypertension, symptoms of goitre are far commoner in those people who know that they have a goitre. The commonest of these are:

(1) a feeling of pressure in the throat
(2) choking sensations
(3) a lump in the throat
(4) difficulty in swallowing
(5) difficulty in breathing

Collectively these symptoms can be referred to as globus hystericus or more appropriately today as a thyroid neurosis. When such symptoms are referable to a goitre the goitre is large or retrosternal. Usually goitre is asymptomatic – the patient notices it herself or someone else does so. Here the unstated fear is often of cancer which needs to be dealt with – one reason why follow-up without investigation and with a worried expression is not advised. Other symptoms that occur in goitre are:

(1) Pain – *generalized* in subacute thyroiditis, auto-immune or viral, infiltrating neoplasm especially anaplastic carcinoma or lymphoma; rare pyogenic or granulomatous infiltration;

(2) Pain – *localized* in haemorrhage into a cyst or neoplasm.

Assessment

The most important clinical assessment –a careful examination of the gland – has been emphasized. Other clinical pointers are:

(1) Past history of goitre, hyperthyroidism, thyroid surgery, radioiodine treatment;

(2) Positive family history – this is seen in auto-immune thyroiditis, Graves's disease and dyshormonogenetic goitres;

(3) Careful drug screen – for antithyroid drugs and dietary and chemotherapeutic goitrogens and thyroid hormone replacement and oestrogens;

(4) Past history of pernicious anaemia – this means that auto-immune thyroiditis is more likely.

Investigations

Those which are useful and available are:

(1) X-ray of neck
(2) thyroid function tests
(3) thyroid auto-antibodies
(4) TRH testing
(5) thyroid scan
(6) thyroid ultrasound
(7) specialized tests

The place of each test can be summarized as follows below, in terms of indications, information provided and contraindications.

Neck X-ray

This investigation:

(1) Is useful in large goitres, longstanding multinodular goitres and goitres where retrosternal extension is suspected;

(2) May show tracheal compression or deviation (ask for lateral views as well as anterior-posterior); calcification may occur in old haemorrhagic cysts or more diffusely in papillary carcinoma;

(3) Is not indicated in 'simple' goitre'.

Thyroid function tests

(1) These are indicated in all cases of goitre since minor degrees of hypo and hyperthyroidism cannot be detected clinically.

(2) Different thyroid function tests have different sensitivities for the detection of different thyroid diseases.

Routinely a serum total thyroxine (T4) concentration is the best test. In addition if hypothyroidism is suspected – request a serum TSH. If hyperthyroidism is suspected request a serum total tri-iodothyramine (T3) concentration. This is particularly valuable when the goitre is nodular.

Thyroid function tests can be difficult to interpret – see Table 3 for examples.

Thyroid autoantibodies

Antibodies occur that are directed against thyroglobulin (usually detected by the tanned red cell test) and against thyroid micro-somes – cytoplasmic antibodies usually detected by a complement fixation test. These antibodies occur in the general population; about 6% of women and 2% of men will have either type of antibody but less than 1% will have both. In thyroid disease these antibodies are found in those conditions of auto-immune origin:

(1) Hashimoto's thyroiditis subacute and chronic: high titres;

(2) The atrophic form of thyroiditis giving myxoedema: lower titres;

(3) Graves's disease: 85% usually low titre.

Request this test in the presence of a diffuse or multinodular goitre when auto-immune thyroid disease is suspected.

The test is particularly helpful in:

(1) The diagnosis of Hashimoto's thyroiditis; high titres of both type of antibody are usually found;

(2) The exclusion of Hashimoto's thyroiditis in a patient with a firm or hard diffusely enlarged gland or a family history;

(3) The definition of a group of patients with Graves's disease and 'active' auto-immune thyroiditis; high titres may mean the patient will develop hypothyroidism.

Table 3   Abnormal thyroid function tests seen in a variety of clinical conditions

Clinical condition	Serum T4 level	Serum T3 level	T3 resin uptake	Serum TSH level	Clinical thyroid state
T3 toxicosis	normal (N)	↑	↑ or N	N	Toxic
On oestrogens or pregnancy. High thyroxine binding globulins in blood. This is also seen as a normal variant.	↑N↓	↑ or N	↓	N	Euthyroid
Sick euthyroid severe non-thyroidal illness	↑N↓	↓	N	N	Euthyroid
Compensated euthyroid seen on antithyroid drugs or early in the development of hypothyroidism	N↓	↓↑	N	↑	Euthyroid
After iodide administration	↑↓	↓↑	↓N	N↑	Usually euthyroid, could be hypo or toxic
Starvation anorexia nervosa	N	→↓	N	N	Euthyroid
On amiodarone	↓	→↓	N	N↓	Euthyroid
On lithium	N↓	N↑	N	N↓	Euthyroid, hypo
On β-adrenergic blockers	N	N↓	N	N	Euthyroid
Hepatic failure	→↓	→↓	N↓	N	Euthyroid
Renal failure	N↓	→↓	N↓	N	Euthyroid
On phenytoin salicylates Heparin	N↓	N↓	N	N	Euthyroid

There are no real contraindications, but low titre non-specific results are found in a variety of thyroid diseases. The test is not usually helpful in multinodular goitre or single adenoma of the gland.

TRH testing

This test is done by injecting intravenously 200 μg of thyrotrophin releasing hormone (TRH). A basal specimen and specimens at 20 and 60 minutes are taken for TSH estimation.

The test is of no clinical benefit in clearcut cases of either hyper- or hypothyroidism.

Thyroid scan

Thyroid scanning is now routinely carried out using isotopically labelled ^{99m}Tc pertechnetate which is trapped by the thyroid similarly to iodine. The radioactive dose received by the patient is smaller as the half-life is only 6 hours.

(1) The indications are: all asymmetrical goitres, single nodules, most multinodular goitres unless known to be stable, and rapid increase in size or abnormal 'suspect' features in a diffuse goitre.

(2) The important benefits are the classification of nodules as 'cold' (not taking up isotope) or 'hot' (taking up isotope). Most malignancies of the thyroid occur in 'cold' areas. Single nodules of the gland producing thyrotoxicosis ('hot' nodules) present differently, often with T3 toxicosis, and are treated differently.

(3) The test is not usually of help in uncomplicated diffuse goitres.

Thyroid ultrasound

This is usually carried out with scanning.

(1) It is of greatest help in defining a 'cold' area on scan as solid (i.e. malignancy likely) or cystic (malignancy less likely).
(2) It is not to be interpreted as ruling out malignancy.

Specialized tests

There are many specialized tests for the thyroidologist but the following are worth a mention, so that the GP knows of their existence:

(1) T3 suppression tests – still useful for the exclusion or definition of autonomous thyroid hormone secretion by nodules,

(2) Perchlorate discharge test – useful in the diagnosis of dyshormonogenetic goitres,

(3) TSH receptor binding activity – a new name for the very similar kind of tests known as LATS, LATSP, TsAb, TSI, which are associated with thyroid stimulating immunoglobulin activity found in Graves's disease.

Management

'Simple goitre'

In most cases a small diffuse goitre requires no treatment except reassurance. As the patient (who may have discovered 'the lump' herself) may well be worried about cancer it is important *not* to alarm the patient by overzealous investigation of trivial goitre but to judge *effectively* which require further investigation and treatment and which do not. Proceed as follows:

(1) Goitre identified,
(2) Assess for suspect features as indicated above,
(3) Obtain thyroid function tests on all cases,

(4) Goitre suspect, large, thyroid hormone status abnormality present or not sure – *Refer* or manage as indicated,

(5) Simple diffuse small goitre, no suspect features, thyroid function tests normal – reassure.

It is probably unwise to tell the patient that she has a goitre before being in a position to reassure her that it is 'simple' or all is well or that the gland is functioning normally, unless you plan to refer or investigate further.

Hyperthyroidism and hypothyroidism

Manage these conditions as indicated in the separate sections dealing with them, below.

Therapy with thyroxine

Suppression therapy with thyroxine is given most effectively for dyshormonogenetic goitre and drug or goitrogen induced goitre. In auto-immune thyroiditis it is worth trying to reduce the size of the gland *where this large* even though the patient is apparently euthyroid. In longstanding goitre or when there is a multinodular goitre this treatment is rarely effective. Goitres that occur at puberty or in pregnancy are usually soft, small and diffuse. Reassurance is all that is usually required but T4 therapy will usually shrink them. Whenever thyroxine therapy is given the dosage should be monitored with serum levels to keep within the normal range.

Surgical therapy

Surgical therapy for goitre is indicated where:

(1) There is a suspicion of malignancy on clinical grounds already mentioned followed by the finding of a 'cold' area on scan. The extent of surgery will depend on the findings. For a

definite thyroid cancer it will consist of radical thyroidectomy possibly with neck dissection; an attempt to remove all thyroid tissue; for a solid 'cold' nodule with dubious histology a hemithyroidectomy may suffice.

(2) There are pressure symptoms from tracheal compression or large goitre.

(3) There is a major cosmetic problem.

The typical clinical course and assessment of a thyroid malignancy are shown in Table 4.

Table 4   Clinical course and assessments of a thyroid malignancy

Typical clinical course of a thyroid malignancy	Factors usually involved in assessment
Clinical suspicion of malignancy	Rapid size increase or new symptoms in an asymmetrical or nodular gland. *Urgent referral*
Thyroid scan shows cold area; and/or ultrasound shows solid	Thyroid status is assessed simultaneously – usually euthyroid – hyperthyroid is against cancer. Multinodular glands are rarely malignant. 10–20% of 'cold' nodules are malignant.
Surgical removal: if possible	Correct thyroid status if necessary before surgery Extent of surgery varies.
Thyroid cancer regime	Precise treatment depends on histology

Thyroid cancer regimes

For undifferentiated thyroid neoplasms, secondary infiltration of the thyroid and medullary carcinoma of the thyroid, the treatment is radical surgery, possibly with radiotherapy.

Lymphoma of the thyroid is treated as other stage IV lymphomas. For differentiated thyroid neoplasm – papillary or follicular carcinoma, – the treatment is radical surgery. After this a state of hypothyroidism is induced by withdrawal of T4 replacement therapy. This induces further differentiation so that the cancer will take up radioiodine. A large dose of radioiodine (150 mCi) is administered to destroy all differentiated thyroid tissue. This process of induced hypothyroidism followed by total body scanning to detect residual radioiodine trapping tissue followed by therapy doses of radioiodine is then repeated until all tumour is destroyed. The prognosis is reasonably good.

Symptoms

The greatest need for symptomatic treatment is in relation to thyroid neurosis:

(1) First and foremost is not to aid development of neurosis by focussing attention on a trivial goitre, particularly as an explanation for throat symptoms that you already consider are really due to anxiety.

(2) Once developed give reasoned assurance with the information that the symptoms are very commonly due to worry and the goitre *is not cancerous* and is demonstrably not causing any obstruction. People are not reassured when required to attend for frequent follow-up examinations 'to see if it is growing', though yearly review of multinodular goitre for cosmetic assessment is justifiable after investigation.

Information to patient and family

(1) Goitres affect 10% of the population and are much commoner in females.

(2) Most goitres are entirely safe and after assessment are best forgotten about.

(3) A small percentage of goitres do require further investigation after which a clear prognosis can be given.

(4) A very small number require operation (for obstruction, cosmetic reasons and neoplasm).

(5) Some goitres do run in families.

Prevention

Now that household salt and bread are iodized the major goitre prevention measure against iodine deficiency in Britain has been taken.

After care

It is important to preserve a balance between effective after care and too intensive follow-up with attendant anxiety.

(1) Autoimmune thyroiditis – yearly examination and thyroid function tests both before and after T4 replacement is given. People can become hypothyroid at any time.

(2) Hyper- and hypothyroidism – see the relevant sections, below.

(3) Multinodular goitre – after investigation has excluded neoplasm and obstruction and the patient is known to be euthyroid, review yearly when large.

(4) Viral thyroiditis – thyroid function tests repeated at increasing intervals for 2 years.

(5) Those of T4 replacement – see the hypothyroidism section.

(6) Post-surgery – thyroid cancer follow-up as indicated; always check thyroid function and serum calcium level 1 month and 8 months after surgery.

HYPOTHYROIDISM

What is it?

Hypothyroidism exists when the thyroid gland fails to produce enough thyroid hormone to maintain the body in perfect health. It is extremely common, affecting around 1% of the community, is still underdiagnosed, particularly in the elderly, and causes a great deal of ill health. It is commoner in women, tends to run in families, can appear at any time of life and is often referred to as myxoedema – an unsatisfactory term, as this one feature may not be present or not be noticeable in milder cases. The causes of hypothyroidism are auto-immune thyroiditis (goitrous, 'Hashimoto's disease' and atrophic forms), exposure to radioiodine or antithyroid drugs or dietary goitrogens, thyroidectomy, replacement of thyroid tissue by inflammatory tissue, granuloma or neoplasm including viral or De Quervain's thyroiditis, and congenital absence hypoplasia or ectopia of the thyroid gland. In addition, pituitary failure causes a hypothyroidism.

What problems?

(1) Very high prevalence means one should always be on the look-out for this condition. It also contributes to the considerable follow-up problems.

(2) The condition is often missed particularly in its milder forms (borderline hypothyroidism) where clinical features are less dramatic.

(3) It has insidious onset – auto-immune thyroid disease predisposes to the development of hypothyroidism which may supervene at any time.

(4) Long term monitoring of replacement therapy is necessary, giving a large patient load; 15% of treated patients with hypothyroidism will stop taking replacement therapy.

Clinical features

Hypothyroidism may be clinically gross or clinically undetectable or anywhere between the two. The important thing is to ask yourself of any state of poorly defined ill health – could this be hypothyroidism?

Overt hypothyroidism

The classical clinical description of mental and physical slowing, cold intolerance, constipation, dry hair and skin, weight gain, muscular aches and pains, tingling hands (carpal tunnel syndrome), croaky voice, facial puffiness and pallor, watering eyes and menorrhagia and mental change does not prevent this condition from being frequently missed.

(1)   Very often the onset is so insidious the patient, her family and the doctor do not notice the changes developing.

(2)   Specific complaints may not be made – the 'classical features' appearing in the patient's conversation as a series of non-specific grumbles.

(3)   People may not complain of the cold; they put on extra clothes.

(4)   Always think of hypothyroidism as a possibility in the assessment of a patient with any of the specific complaints mentioned above and particularly with depression.

Borderline hypothyroidism

Symptoms are mild and often single; tiredness, puffy eyes or dry skin may occur. It is usually not possible to be clinically confident of the diagnosis. Very often a family history of thyroid disease or the presence of, say, pernicious anaemia can help to raise the index of suspicion.

In most cases of possible hypothyroidism, slowing of the relaxation phase of the reflexes occurs and this can be a valuable sign.

However, the clinical evaluation of hypothyroidism is far less sensitive than thyroid function tests which should be requested whenever the clinical suspicion has been raised (Table 5).

Table 5   Assessment of hypothyroidism

---

(1)   Bring the condition to the front of your mind. One tactic is to ask yourself 'Is this hypothyroidism' for all ill-defined health, problems *including those in children*

(2)   Look for specific features – puffy pale face, dry skin, delayed reflexes, goitre

(3)   If any clinical suspicions arise proceed directly to thyroid function tests and autoantibodies

(4)   Remember T4 may be normal; TSH is always raised, but a raised TSH is not necesarily specific of hypothyroidism. A normal TSH excludes hypothyroidism not due to pituitary disease

---

Assessment and investigation

In assessment of hypothyroidism the first prerequisite is to think of the condition. In severe cases the clinical picture will then 'fall into place'. In borderline hypothyroidism one cannot be sure clinically and it is best to proceed immediately to thyroid function tests. Prolonged clinical pondering is not of value.

(1)   A serum T4 level is not sensitive enough to pick up all cases who will benefit from thyroid hormone replacement. Many borderline cases have a serum T4 within the normal range.

(2)   A serum TSH level will be elevated in all cases of hypothyroidism due to thyroid disease (i.e. not those due to pituitary failure). However, some patients are able to maintain the euthyroid state by elevating TSH and do not benefit from thyroid hormone replacement. This is called 'compensated euthyroidism'.

(3)   Autoantibody tests are of value because the identification of auto-immune thyroiditis allows definition of an at-risk patient. A positive family history or presence of other auto-immune disease such as pernicious anaemia can also serve the same function. Any patient who has ever received radioiodine treatment for hyperthyroidism is at risk of developing hypothyroidism for life.

(4)   If goitre is present assess as previously indicated.

(5)   A TRH test showing an exaggerated response of serum TSH is of value in borderline cases and sometimes in assessing the adequacy of replacement therapy.

(6)   A blood count should be routine once hypothyroidism has been identified, because anaemia (often macrocytic) is common and there may be coexisting megaloblastic anaemia due to pernicious anaemia.

(7)   Exclusion of pituitary disease. In hypothyroidism of pituitary origin the skin is usually fine, not coarse, and paler than in hypothyroidism due to thyroid disease. There is almost always amenorrhoea and absence of axillary or pubic hair. There may be a history of postpartum haemorrhage or evidence of an intracranial space occupying lesion (headache – visual field loss). When in doubt request a lateral skull film as most cases of pituitary failure occur in association with a pituitary tumour.

Hypothyroidism in children

In the newborn the earlier the diagnosis of congenital hypothyroidism the better. The child may have a full-blown picture with puffy skin, large protruding tongue, umbilical hernia and delayed reflexes but the diagnosis should be considered in any child who fails to thrive or is sluggish. Neonatal jaundice may be prolonged, offering a further clue. Cord blood can now be screened to detect this condition. In the older child there is retarded growth with delayed and deformed epiphyses on X-ray – epiphyseal dysgenesis. The arms and legs are characteristically short. Milder degrees of juvenile hypothyroidism may not have severe mental deficiency as in the complete congenital variety – characteristically some thyroid tissue, often as a lingual or other ectopic thyroid, is functional. In still older children (teenagers) the features of juvenile hypothyroidism approximate to the adult state. Thyroid function tests are diagnostic, but X-rays to assess epiphyseal maturity should also be requested in investigation.

The ultimate investigation, particularly in borderline hypothyroidism, is a therapeutic trial with T4 to see if the patient's symptoms are relieved. If they are not, stop the T4.

Management

Specific

The therapy of choice is thyroxine (T4). There is no place for thyroid extract and almost no place for therapy with T3.

(1) In young people it is customary to start with 50–100 μg a day and after several weeks increase to 100–200 μg, the expected replacement dose. There is no need for undue haste in correcting metabolic abnormalities that have been present for a long time but similarly one need not exercise undue caution in increasing the dose.

(2) In elderly people it is wise to proceed with smaller increments of 50 μg at monthly intervals as there is a danger of precipitating ischaemic heart disease.

(3) In those with symptomatic ischaemic heart disease, extreme caution is necessary when increasing the dose of thyroxine. It is often not possible to render such patients euthyroid. Simultaneous β-adrenergic-blockade is probably dangerous and should be done only by those experienced in such regimens. There is some place for therapy with T3 which has a shorter half-life than T4 so it is possible to reduce the effects more quickly.

The most important thing in the chronic management of all patients with hypothyroidism on T4 is that the serum levels of thyroid hormone achieved by therapy are measured routinely and dosage is adjusted until the patient is euthyroid. Serum TSH levels and TRH testing can be of help here, and there are some caveats:

(1) Always allow sufficient time (at least 2 weeks) for equilibrium to be established before checking the effect on T4 levels of a dosage increment.

(2) Warn the patient that if chest pain supervenes they should drop back to the previous dose.

(3) Resist the temptation to raise and lower the dosage of T4 on symptoms without blood tests.

Symptomatic management

(1) On adequate replacement therapy, symptoms that the patient has learnt are thyroid-related (cold intolerance, palpitations, etc) are probably due to anxiety but are not due to 'the thyroid'. Dosage should be altered on blood tests.

(2) Many patients complain of 'new problems' after treatment with T4 has been started – which is often disappointing to the doctor, expecting that the patient on her first return after treatment will be greatly improved. This state of affairs is probably due to increased alertness and articulation on the patient's part in noticing problems which she had previously ignored.

(3) Carpal tunnel syndrome usually improves but may take a year or more if nerve damage has occurred. Surgery is still sometimes needed.

(4) Haematinics are not required for the anaemia. If it does not respond to T4, suspect complicating iron deficiency or pernicious anaemia.

Information to patient/family

(1) T4 is not a drug but a normal bodily constituent. It does not affect pregnancy.

(2) The importance of taking tablets regularly on an empty stomach must be stressed, together with the importance of monitoring blood levels to establish correct dose and then (yearly) to maintain therapy correctly.

(3) The thyroxine replaces that which their thyroid gland would produce if it was functioning.

(4) Once therapy (other than a trial of T4) is started it is for life replacement not cure.

(5) Thyroid disease does run in families but is not dangerous if detected and correctly treated.

(6) There is no danger if T4 tablets are accidentally omitted for a few days (unlike steroids). Symptoms are unlikely to supervene for a week or so, in fact.

Prevention

There is little we can do to prevent hypothyroidism except:

(1) that due to antithyroid drugs,

(2) possibly that due to radioiodine therapy.

Efforts should be aimed at early detection.

After care

After care is best carried out by the general practitioner. Patients with hypothyroidism should be on an at-risk register and be periodically reviewed. Once the correct dose of T4 has been established a yearly review with T4 and TSH levels is satisfactory.

HYPERTHYROIDISM

What is it?

The term hyperthyroidism is used synonymously with thyrotoxicosis to describe the syndrome resulting from the exposure of body tissues to excess thyroid hormone. There are many causes.

(1) Graves' disease or toxic diffuse goitre: auto-immune in origin due to presence of abnormal thyroid-stimulating immunoglobulins. Endocrine exophthalmos only occurs in Graves' disease. Also pre-tibial myxoedema and thyroid acropachy occur;

(2) Toxic multinodular goitre; of unknown cause: autonomous hyperfunction of multiple nodules;

(3) Toxic single adenoma ('hot nodule') : autonomous hyperfunction in a single adenoma of the gland;

(4) Thyrotoxicosis factitia (due to exogenous thyroid hormone);

(5) Jod–Basedow phenomenon (iodide induced hyperthyroidism);

(6) Struma ovarii (ovarian tumour secreting thyroid hormone);

(7) Production of TSH by tumours;

(8) Transient neonatal hyperthyroidism seen in the newborn offspring of women with Graves' disease.

All causes of hyperthyroidism that result from thyroid pathology are commoner in women. The condition may occur at all ages from the newborn to the very elderly. Hyperthyroidism is very common, with a prevalance of almost 1% in the community. There is a familial tendency and in Graves' disease a relationship to other thyroid auto-immune disease and genetic factors as shown by HLA typing.

What problems?

In terms of problems we refer mainly to causes (1) – (3), above.

Occasionally patients take thyroid hormone to aid weight loss etc, but most cases of factitious thyrotoxicosis are due to over-treatment of hypothyroidism by the doctor, which is common. The remaining causes of hyperthyroidism are all rare. Jod–Basedow phenomenon occurs in iodine-deficient areas where there is almost ubiquitous multinodular goitre. Introduction of iodine into the diet can cause hyperthyroidism. The same phenomenon which is due to loss of thyroidal autoregulatory mechanisms for iodine can occur in single and multiple 'hot nodules' in non-iodine-deficient areas.

Problems for the three common clinical causes of hyperthyroidism are:

(1)   The condition is extremely common causing large patient loads,

(2)   Though diagnosis in typical cases is not difficult there is an extremely wide range of 'unusual' presentations and clinical assessment is inferior to laboratory tests,

(3)   No method of treatment is uniformly successful,

(4)   The condition tends to be chronic and relapsing and therefore often needs monitoring for long periods of time,

(5)   In Graves' disease problems with the eyes, skin and also in newborn infants occur.

Clinical features

Graves' disease is the commonest cause of hyperthyroidism, followed by toxic multinodular goitre and then toxic single adenoma (about 10% of cases of hyperthyroidism).

(1)   The classical presentation of *Graves' disease* is a woman aged 20–40 with nervous irritability, excess sweating, heat

intolerance, palpitations and weight loss with a good appetite. On examination there is hyperkinesis – a jerky restless choreiform state, warm moist hands, tachycardia and fine tremor.

(2)   The presence of exophthalmos and a large diffuse goitre often alert the doctor to the presence of Graves' disease. Both may be absent, however, and the presence of either does not indicate that there is current hyperthyroidism, merely that the patient has Graves' disease, in which the presence of hyperthyroidism is not constant.

(3)   Treatment with β-adrenergic blockers can mask most of the clinical features of hyperthyroidism.

(4)   The presentation in elderly patients is different. Atrial fibrillation is common and may be the sole abnormality. In general, the cardiovascular system takes the brunt of the disorder in older people. Unexplained cardiac failure, recurrent paroxysmal tachydysrhythmias and resistance to the action of digoxin are indications for thyroid function testing.

(5)   A variety of atypical presentations occur including weight loss and depression without hyperexcitability (apathetic hyperthyroidism); myopathy; diarrhoea; abnormal behaviour; mood change.

(6)   The eyes. A clear rim of sclera above and below the cornea in the position of horizontal gaze indicates exophthalmos. Periorbital puffiness and aching watery eyes with conjunctival oedema are other positive clues to the ophthalmopathy of Graves' disease. Lid lag may occur due to sympathomimetic overactivity in any thyrotoxic or anxious patient. Where exophthalmos is present check that the patient can close both eyes fully. If the patient cannot, corneal abrasion may occur. In malignant exophthalmos the optic nerve is endangered and visual acuity drops. This condition requires immediate referral. The ophthalmopathy of Graves' disease can be unilateral. Eye signs do not indicate that hyperthyroidism is present.

(7) Other auto-immune phenomena – periostitis, pretibial myxoedema and finger clubbing (thyroid acropachy) – also occur in Graves' disease.

(8) In *toxic multinodular goitre* the patient is generally a little older. There are no eye signs or skin changes. The goitre may be large or small but is nodular clinically and on scanning. It may be impossible to distinguish clinically from Graves' disease without exophthalmos where prolonged thyroid stimulation has induced nodular change. The hyperthyroidism is less likely to remit spontaneously or by use of antithyroid drug therapy.

(9) In *toxic single adenoma* there are no eye signs and very often no obvious goitre. Examine the gland carefully for atrophy of the opposite lobe and a swelling limited to the midline. Clinical features may mislead with a high incidence of anxiety, depression and apathetic hyperthyroidism.

(10) The presence of a true thyroid bruit in a patient who has not been on antithyroid drugs for 2 months and who has not got a dyshormonogenetic goitre is a strong indication of the presence of hyperthyroidism.

Table 6   Unusual clinical presentations of hyperthyroidism

(1) Weight loss and depression (apathetic hyperthyroidism)

(2) Lone atrial fibrillation in the elderly

(3) Unexplained cardiac failure or paroxysmal dysrhythmias

(4) Myopathy

(5) Diarrhoea

(6) Abnormal behaviour

(7) Mood change

(11) Myopathy usually affecting the shoulder girdle muscles is very common in hyperthyroidism, is often missed clinically and is a useful confirmatory sign (Table 6).

Assessment

As in hypothyroidism, the clinical assessment of hyperthyroidism is inferior to thyroid function tests. Once the possibility of hyperthyroidism has occurred to you, request thyroid function tests. However, the precise cause of the patient's hyperthyroidism is in many cases just as important as its presence. Careful examination of the thyroid gland is again the important and often neglected procedure – is there a diffuse goitre, a multinodular goitre, a single nodule or no visible or palpable thyroid tissue? The cause of hyperthyroidism affects the management.

Also be sure to:

(1) assess cardiac function and rhythm,

(2) assess the degree of myopathy,

(3) assess the condition of the eyes.

Investigations

The best single routine thyroid function test in the assessment of hyperthyroidism is the serum total T3. If serum T4 is routinely used then T3-toxicosis may be missed. The corresponding T4-toxicosis – where serum T4 is elevated but serum T3 is normal – is much rarer than T3-toxicosis. Twelve per cent of patients with Graves' disease have T3-toxicosis, but the distinction gains paramount importance in the assessment of toxic single adenoma where 50% of patients present with T3-toxicosis.

(1) The TRH test is useful in doubtful or borderline cases where a flat or unresponsive test confirms and a responsive test excludes the diagnosis.

(2)   Remember that a raised serum T4 level (or even a raised serum T3 level) can be caused by an elevated thyroxine binding globulin concentration (TBG). This is the protein in the blood chiefly responsible for the carriage of thyroid hormones. The level of this protein is raised by oestrogens but a high level can occur familiarly or sporadically on a congenital basis.

(3)   Always enquire for oral oestrogen use or possibility of pregnancy when assessing hyperthyroidism.

(4)   TBG levels can now be measured directly in serum but the resin uptake test is still widely used to identify this problem. In hyperthyroidism both the T4 level and the resin test are raised. In hypothyroidism both are low. In elevated TBG states the T4 level is high but the resin test is low. The T4 value can be multiplied by the resin test results to provide a free thyroxine index (FTI) which remains within the normal range in abnormal TBG states (Figure 7).

(5)   The ultimate tests for hyperthyroidism are raised values for the free thyroid hormones – a raised free T4 and above all a raised free T3. This testing can be done in most large hospitals nowadays by arrangement.

Management

The aims of management in hyperthyroidism are to:

(1)   Render the patient euthyroid,

(2)   Allow metabolic recovery to occur so that wasted muscles recover and normal weight is regained,

(3)   Prevent recurrence,

(4)   Detect recurrence early when it does occur,

(5)   Achieve all of the above whilst maintaining the person's total physical, psychological and social health.

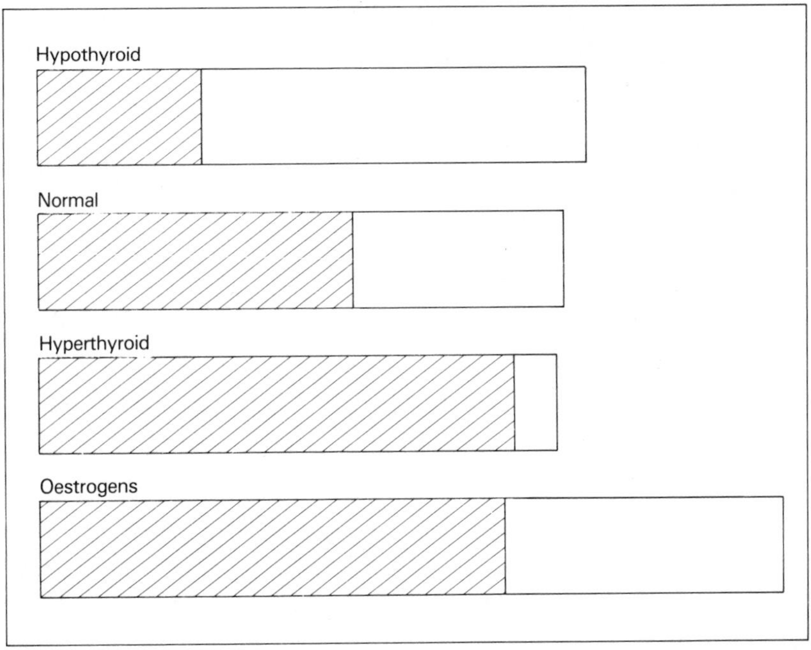

Figure 7 Relationships between saturation of TBG and resin uptake test result. Columns indicate TBG levels; hatched areas represent serum T4 levels; blank areas of the column indicate TBG free of bound T4 and able to compete with resin for radio-labelled T3 added in the resin test procedure. The lower this 'spare TBG capacity', the higher is the resin uptake value and vice versa.

Specific

There are three main treatments for hyperthyroidism although, as will be seen, they are often used in combination to fulfil the aims of treatment. There are also some less important measures that will be discussed. The generally used treatments are:

(1)   antithyroid drugs
(2)   surgery
(3)   radioiodine

and in addition we consider the place of:

(4)   β-adrenergic blockers
(5)   iodine.

Antithyroid drugs

The commonly used drugs are as follows:

(1)   Carbimazole (neomercazole); initial dose 30–45 mg; minimum 5 mg per day.

(2)   Propylthiouracil (PTU) which also has a secondary extrathyroidal action in preventing the conversion of T4 to T3; initial dose 400 mg; minimum 25 mg per day.

(3)   Potassium perchlorate which acts as a competitive blocker of iodide in the thyroidal iodide trap mechanism; initial dose 600–800 mg; minimum 200 mg per day. DO NOT give iodides to patients controlled on the drug.

In Britain carbimazole (CMZ) is the drug most commonly used. It is a very safe drug despite a fairly long list of side-effects including:

(1)   agranulocytosis
(2)   skin rashes
(3)   jaundice
(4)   hair loss
(5)   fever with lymphadenopathy
(6)   a polyarteritis nodosa syndrome

It is also a very effective and very cheap drug. The regimes to be described are for CMZ. PTU may be used when people are allergic to CMZ. Potassium perchlorate can be used synergistically with either CMZ or PTU in those people whose hyperthyroidism does not respond to high doses of these drugs. This is unusual – CMZ has a cumulative action and increasing the dose too quickly can lead to profound hypothyroidism later. The side-effects of PTU and perchlorate are similar to CMZ but a little more common. Aplastic anaemia and nephrosis may occur with perchlorate.

Use of CMZ

Measure the white blood cell count (w.b.c.) always before starting CMZ therapy to exclude pre-existing problems. Routine w.b.c. on therapy are not justified. CMZ is used in almost every case of hyperthyroidism to render the patient euthyroid. Thus it is given alone, before surgery and often before radioiodine therapy also. There is also no point in operating on a patient who is wasted, weak and not in ideal circumstances to face an operation simply because the serum thyroid hormone values are normal. Thus antithyroid drugs are often used to fulfil the second aim of allowing metabolic recovery. There is some evidence that antithyroid drugs, by acting on the lymphocytes within the thyroid gland which produce thyroid stimulating antibodies, may also help to prevent recurrence and fulfil the third aim of therapy, but there is no doubt that destructive therapies do this better. Nevertheless, despite the fact that 50% of people with Graves' disease will relapse after a course of CMZ, this therapy is used alone in the majority of cases. This is because:

(1) Many people do not want an operation,
(2) Many people do not want a scar,
(3) Surgery may be contraindicated,
(4) A sufficiently experienced thyroid surgeon may not be available,
(5) Surgery is best avoided in certain groups:
    children
    pregnancy
    those with small goitres who are less likely to relapse
(6) Around 50% of people will not relapse and are better treated without operation.

When CMZ is used alone as the sole intended treatment then one or the other of the two methods shown should be used, but not a mixture of them both.

Titration partially blocks the gland to produce normal thyroid hormone levels. The second regime keeps the gland completely blocked and T4 is given in addition (Table 7).

Table 7 Regimes with carbimazole (CMZ)

Titration	*Block and Supplement*
Start 30–45 mg per day	Choose patients who will be able to comply with a more complicated regime
Review in 4 weeks	
Lower the dose when evidence of a response is obtained	Explain the rationale
Lower the dose incrementally to 5–15 mg per day	Start 45 mg per day
	See in 4 weeks
Be guided by clinical findings plus thyroid hormone levels remembering (1) when they were done (2) the likely time course projection of changes already noted	Do not add T4 until clear evidence of response is obtained
	Add a full replacement dose of T4
	Do not lower CMZ to below 30 mg a day
	Check T4 levels achieved
See at least monthly throughout 6–24 months	Once controlled you may see less frequently (8-week intervals)
	6–24 months

DON'T MIX
Do not end up with a patient who is poorly controlled on a half-dose of CMZ and a half-supplement of T4

Remember that:

(1) CMZ can be given in a once daily dose or in divided doses;

(2) Thyroid function tests are difficult to interpret on CMZ since the blocked gland secretes less T4 and more T3. Also, CMZ has a cumulative action and tests may be out of date. Use a combination of tests and clinical judgements of response such as weight gain, symptom scores and *watch the gland;*

(3) CMZ should be given for at least 6 months to 2 years;

(4) CMZ should not be stopped abruptly.

When to stop CMZ

(1) In general give for at least 6 months and preferably a year.

(2) A gland that gets smaller or loses a bruit is a good index of remission.

(3) A gland that gets larger or gains a bruit may be overtreated. Check and change to 'block and supplement' if necessary.

(4) Thyroid autoantibody titres plus HLA typing may be able to predict those who are likely to relapse. A combination of high titres and HLA-B8 positivity is suggestive. Similar claims have been made for lack of T3 suppressibility and short duration of therapy.

(5) Always tail off CMZ – never stop abruptly.

Management plans in hyperthyroidism

(1) First render the patient euthyroid.

(2) Next discuss the treatment options with the patient in depth.

(3) State the management plan – for instance a plan suitable for most Graves' disease patients in the first instance could be 'treat with CMZ for 1 year'.

For recurrent Graves' disease or toxic multinodular goitre the plan could be 'render euthryroid, return to health, then surgery', or 'render euthyroid, then radioiodine at leisure'.

For mild cases in the elderly or single toxic adenoma, a suitable plan could be 'radioiodine directly'.

Surgery

Surgery is a very effective treatment for hyperthyroidism. It may be used in the following circumstances:

(1) Some people with Graves' disease for the first time who prefer surgery,

(2) Recurrent Graves' disease, particularly with large glands,

(3) Toxic multinodular goitre,

(4) Toxic single adenoma.

Surgery in Graves' disease carries a much lower relapse rate (around 10%) than CMZ therapy alone. The mortality is less than 1% and the morbidity is not high. Risks of postoperative recurrent laryngeal nerve damage and hypoparathyroidism are slight in experienced hands. Hypothyroidism develops more commonly after surgery in those with high autoantibody titres.

In toxic multinodular goitre surgery is the treatment of choice when the goitre is large, provided there are no contraindications. In toxic single adenoma the removal of the 'hot' nodule provides a permanent cure.

Radioiodine therapy

Indications are:

(1) The frail or elderly,

(2) Relapsing Graves' disease or multinodular goitre post surgery,

(3) Toxic single adenoma.

What problems?

(1) The possible development of thyroid cancer is not now considered to be a risk of radioiodine treatment.

(2) The fact that persons who have received radioiodine treatment are at risk of developing hypothyroidism for the remainder of their lives, however, still limits the use of this treatment in young people. Those who have received radioiodine must be followed-up for life.

72

(3) It is difficult to provide the dose that will render the patient euthyroid with minimal risk of relapsing hyperthyroidism or development of hypothyroidism in the months after a therapy dose. Some centres adopt an 'ablative' approach in which the thyroid is purposefully destroyed. The patient is then put on T4 replacement therapy (but still must be followed-up – see above).

(4) The therapy must not be given when there is a risk of concurrent pregnancy.

β-Adrenergic blockers

Indications for use are as a short term measure to limit symptoms (particularly palpitations) in newly diagnosed patients. Withdraw the drug as the CMZ takes effect. Use a long acting preparation, say atenolol 50 mg o.m. (very effective in the now rare thyroid storm).

What problems?

(1) Use of β-adrenergic blockers only controls some of the clinical features of hyperthyroidism – acting in the peripheral tissues. It is not a complete therapy and has no effect on the thyroid gland.

(2) β-adrenergic blockers are not to be used to cover surgery in hyperthyroid patients.

Iodine

Inorganic iodide in high doses (over 100 mg per day for some nodular goitres) will acutely inhibit the release of formed thyroid hormone from the gland.

Its uses are as an emergency method to control hyperthyroidism for non-elective surgery, thyroid storm etc.

What problems?

(1) The effect is only temporary (1–3 weeks).

(2) In different dosages iodide may stimulate the gland (*see* Jod–Basedow phenomenon).

(3) Iodide will cause acute hyperthyroidism in a patient controlled on the iodide-trap blocking drug perchlorate.

This is not a therapy for general practice use except in the most extreme emergency.

Symptoms

Symptomatic treatment in hyperthyroidism includes:

(1) β-Adrenergic blockers for palpitations, anxiety, tachycardia,

(2) Digoxin for control of atrial fibrillation (this drug is very ineffective in hyperthyroidism),

(3) Diuretics for cardiac failure induced by hyperthyroidism.

Information to patient/family

(1) Hyperthyroidism is commoner in women and tends to run in families.

(2) It is caused by an overactive thyroid gland. Thyroid hormone in excess causes overactivity and excess energy release as heat.

(3) It is rarely dangerous in the short term but, if left to itself, can damage the heart ultimately.

(4) Therapy is fairly complicated and may take quite a long time. It involves:

    (a) Control of the overactive thyroid gland by tablets. The tablets are very safe but can cause rashes and very occasionally other problems. If you notice a rash or develop a bad sore throat or fever, stop the tablets and see your doctor.

    (b) Restoring normal health.

    (c) Prolonged course of tablets for a year or more, or

    (d) Surgery or radioiodine. Radioiodine is perfectly safe.

(5) It is necessary to see the doctor for some time after treatment has finished to check up on the possibility of recurrence.

(6) There is a small possibility of other members of the family being affected.

(7) There is no specific danger caused by the tablets to the baby in pregnancy but don't try to get pregnant while on the tablets if you can help it, as it makes the management of the condition a little more complicated.

Prevention

Other than careful monitoring of serum levels of thyroid hormone in those on replacement therapy for hypothyroidism to avoid thyrotoxicosis factitia, there is little than can be done in Britain to prevent hyperthyroidism.

After care

It is considerably important that people with hyperthyroidism are monitored closely by the doctor both during and after therapy. The risks are as follows:

(1) The inadequate control of hyperthyroidism on CMZ

(2) Hypothroidism due to CMZ

(3) Relapsing hyperthyroidism after drug therapy
(4) Relapsing hyperthyroidism after radioiodine
(5) Hypothyroidism after radioiodine
(6) Relapsing hyperthyroidism after surgery
(7) Hypothyroidism developing after surgery
(8) Postsurgical hypocalcaemia

Most of the risks have become minimal after a year or so, except post-radioiodine hypothyroidism, which needs lifetime follow-up.

GP and consultant roles

The control of hyperthyroid patients on antithyroid drugs requires considerable experience but there is no reason why it should not be done by the appropriately-trained general practitioner after treatment regimens have been planned at the hospital clinic or jointly. Most of the other follow-up is probably most appropriately done by the general practitioner, leaving the consultant to deal with problems.

Screening tests

These are:

(1) T3 for recurrent hyperthyroidism,

(2) TSH for suspected hypothyroidism.

4
THE PARATHYROID GLAND AND CALCIUM METABOLISM

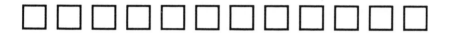

The action of the parathyroid gland cannot be clearly understood without a thorough working knowledge of the metabolism of calcium and appreciation of the interaction between bone, gut, plasma and kidney.

THE PHYSIOLOGY OF BONE PRODUCTION

In normal bone there is a dynamic equilibrium between bone formation and bone resorption. Bone consists of an organic matrix of collagen (osteoid) in which are deposited minerals such as calcium phosphorus and magnesium largely in the form of hydroxyapatite. Bone is formed by osteoblasts which contain a number of enzymes, the most important of which is alkaline phosphatase; this plays a part in bony formation and thus the appearance of bone alkaline phosphatase in the serum can be an indication of osteoblast activity. The control of osteoblast formation is not clearly understood but may be dependent on environmental and mechanical stress. At the same time as bone formation, bone resorption occurs. This is under the control of the osteoclasts which deal with resorption and remodelling. Osteocytes in bone can take up either formative or resorptive functions. Bone resorption and remodelling are under control of parathormone (parathyroid hormone, PTH), vitamin D and thyroxine. If it is appreciated that these two occur in a dynamic relationship then it is easier to understand the pathological changes which occur in association with an overactive or underactive parathyroid gland.

Calcium and phosphorus are essential for healthy bone production and maintenance. They are taken into the diet and stored in the bone. Calcium and phosphorus are also both filtered and actively reabsorbed in the kidney, and calcium is absorbed in the small intestine by an active transport mechanism as well as by diffusion and is re-excreted to the gut. The control of active absorption and excretion is maintained by parathyroid hormone, calcitonin and the analogues of vitamin D. Vitamin D is taken in the diet, being present in egg yolk, fish oils, oily fish and milk. It is also formed by the effect of ultraviolet light on inactive precursors in the skin. Ninety-nine per cent of total body calcium is present in bone. Eighty-five per cent of total body phosphorus is present in bone. Active secretory and reabsorption processes maintain calcium homeostasis between the plasma pool and the bone, the kidney and the gut (Figure 8).

The amounts involved stay fairly constant throughout life, the only exceptions being in the growing child, when more calcium is required for skeletal growth, and in the pregnant woman, when there are more demands both for the fetus and for lactation. A constant concentration of ionized calcium is maintained in the plasma pool, this being essential for efficient neuromuscular function. The total plasma calcium is maintained at 2.2–2.4 mmol/l and about half of this is ionized and physiologically active. Most of the remainder is bound to plasma albumin, the level of which is therefore a powerful determinant of the total plasma calcium level. Always take the plasma albumin level into account when interpreting a plasma calcium value. For every 1 g per litre that the serum albumin falls below 40, add 0.02 mmol/l to the total plasma calcium. The bone calcium store acts as a buffering system to maintain the plasma calcium. The major hormones involved in control of plasma calcium are parathormone and the active component of Vitamin D, which is 1,25-dihydroxycholecalciferol (DHCC). Calcitonin also plays a part. Growth hormone, sex hormones, thyroxine, cortisol and prolactin play a secondary part in the control of calcium metabolism. The physicochemical equilibrium between bone mineral and extracellular fluid is itself sufficient to maintain plasma calcium at up to 2.0 mmol/l.

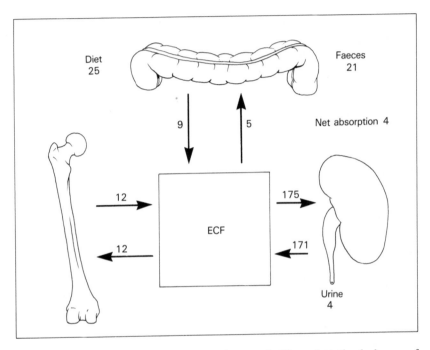

Figure 8 Calcium balance per day in mmol. Note that the balance of bony accretion and resorption is equal and that net absorption from the gut equals the urinary excretion.

Parathormone

The action of parathormone:

(1) Increases the renal tubular resorption of calcium and thus raises the serum calcium,
(2) Decreases the renal threshold for phosphorus,
(3) Increases bone resorption,
(4) Increases active absorption of calcium in gut via 1,25-DHCC.

Increased bone resorption is reflected biochemically by the appearance of more hydroxyproline in the urine due to increased collagen breakdown and a raised alkaline phosphatase in the plasma (secondary to increased formation of bone). Secretion is suppressed when plasma calcium is normal. *Calcitonin* is secreted from the 'C' cells of the thyroid in response to an elevated plasma calcium level. It inhibits bone resorption and decreases tubular reabsorption of phosphate. Parathormone release is stimulated by a fall in the concentration of ionized calcium in the plasma to maintain normal homeostasis.

Vitamin D

Vitamin D is taken in the diet and formed in the skin as cholecalciferol. It is hydroxylated in the liver to form 25-hydroxycholecalciferol (HCC). It is then activated on passage through the kidney to 1,25-DHCC. This acts on gut to mediate the active transport of calcium and on bone to increase the resorption and remineralization of bone. As mentioned before, parathormone appears to be linked in the action of converting 25-HCC to 1,25-DHCC. Hypocalcaemia increases the production of 1,25-DHCC. In the absence of vitamin D the clinical entity of rickets occurs.

RICKETS AND OSTEOMALACIA

What are they?

Rickets occurs in children, osteomalacia in adults. Both conditions are due to vitamin D deficiency. Rickets differs from osteomalacia in that characteristic epiphyseal abnormalities occur in the growing bones. In Britain vitamin D deficiency is quite common, particularly in Asian communities due to a combination of dietary factors and lack of ultraviolet (sun) light. Other at-risk groups are those with malabsorption syndromes and the elderly.

Clinical features

These features are those of hypocalcaemia, as described (below) in the section on hypoparathyroidism. In addition bone pain is very common in osteomalacia, particularly in the pelvis and chest, and widespread muscular weakness is often found. In rickets, skeletal deformities are more common, consisting of genu valgus or varus. The rickety rosary is caused by enlargement of costochondral junctions. In osteomalacia a useful sign is to spring the chest wall or pelvis or wrist, which often elicits tenderness.

Assessment and investigations

Plasma calcium and phosphate levels are both low and the alkaline phosphatase level is raised. This latter investigation is difficult to interpret in children where alkaline phosphatase levels are raised normally above adult values. Radiological abnormalities in rickets consist of widening and deformity of the epiphyseal junctions. In adults with osteomalacia radiological evidence is not as sensitive. There may be generalized rarefaction of the skeleton or characteristic Looser's zones (pseudofractures) may be found, particularly in the pubic rami, ribs and scapulae.

Management

Treat with vitamin D 50 μg daily or 1 β-cholecalciferol 1–2 μg daily. It may take 2 years or more to heal the bones.

After care

Prolonged follow-up and regular monitoring of plasma calcium levels are always mandatory for those receiving vitamin D therapy. At-risk groups should also be followed-up for reassurance.

HYPERFUNCTION AND HYPOFUNCTION

Disorders of parathyroid secretion are mainly divided into hyperfunction and hypofunction.

PRIMARY HYPERPARATHYROIDISM

What is it?

Excess secretion of parathormone from a parathyroid adenoma (75%), hyperplasia of all four parathyroid glands (20%) or a parathyroid carcinoma (5%) result in an increased plasma calcium level. The incidence is as high as 1:1000. The aetiology is unknown. It is more common after the female climacteric. It may be inherited and it may occur in combination with multiple endocrine adenomatosis syndrome. As we have already stated the actions of parathyroid hormone, it follows that the biochemical abnormalities in primary hyperparathyroidism should show an increased plasma calcium and a decreased phosphate, increase in urinary hydroxyproline and an increase in plasma alkaline phosphatase.

Clinical features

(1)   Many cases are asymptomatic, the plasma calcium being found to be elevated incidentally.

(2)   The most common presentation is by renal stones and less commonly by bone pain, pathological fractures or bone cysts. X-rays may show classical osteitis fibrosa cystica but this is becoming uncommon as routine biochemical tests uncover the disease at an earlier stage of its natural history. Subperiosteal resorption of the phalanges is a useful radiological sign. Occasionally those with longstanding hypercalcaemia may develop corneal calcification.

(3)   About 20% of patients get abdominal pain which can be caused by associated peptic ulcer or pancreatitis.

(4) Nephrocalcinosis may lead to hypertension and renal failure.

(5) About the same proportion of patients will present with the symptom complex referable to hypercalcaemia, namely vomiting, thirst, constipation and mental change. The differential diagnosis of hypercalcaemia is shown in Table 8.

Table 8 Common causes of hypercalcaemia

Hyperparathyroidism

Secondary neoplasm ⎰ breast
⎱ bronchus
⎱ kidney

Neoplasms secreting a parathormone-like substance (e.g. bronchus)

Sarcoidosis

Vitamin D intoxication

Immobilization in Paget's disease (seen in thyrotoxicosis and acromegaly)

Milk alkali syndrome (doubtful as a distinct entity)

Assessment and investigation

Biochemical investigations

(1) The plasma calcium is raised in most cases and the plasma phosphate low in about 50%. The alkaline phosphatase is usually normal, being raised only in the minority of patients with significant bone disease.

(2) In general the best approach is to do several estimations of plasma calcium and phosphorus, fasting and without venous occlusion. The low phosphate is helpful as it is generally not seen in other causes of hypercalcaemia.

(3) Serum parathormone estimations are still not as helpful as theoretically they should be.

(4) 24 h urinary calcium excretion may be normal or raised.

Radiological investigation

(1) In most cases diagnosed now radiology is normal.

(2) Always X-ray the hand for subperiosteal erosions.

(3) In occasional cases gross bone disease still occurs with pep-perpot skull, rugger jersey spine, bone cysts and full-blown osteitis fibrosa cystica.

Pathophysiology

The hypercalcaemic clinical picture is frequently missed or incorrectly attributed (it is one cause of thirst, polyuria and weight loss). It is worth understanding the pathophysiology which is as follows:

(1) Hypercalcaemia causes renal tubular damage giving polyuria.

(2) Secondary dehydration causes thirst and constipation (also a neuromuscular effect of hypercalcaemia).

(3) Anorexia, nausea or vomiting exacerbate the dehydration.

(4) A vicious circle is established in which dehydration exacerbates the hypercalcaemia and vice versa.

(It follows that the prime treatment of hypercalcaemia of whatever cause is correction of *dehydration)*.

Management

Surgical removal is the treatment of choice wherever possible. It is advisable to refer only to a surgeon experienced in parathyroid work since location of adenomata can be difficult. Where surgery is not possible, conservative therapy to control hypercalcaemia is possible by ensuring a high fluid intake and by use of oral phosphate therapy. In emergency hypercalcaemia the most important therapy is fluid, usually given as saline intravenously.

After care

It is important to follow-up postsurgical patients for:

(1) recurrent hypercalcaemia
(2) hypocalcaemia
(3) hypertension
(4) renal disease

SECONDARY HYPERPARATHYROIDISM

What is it?

The term is used when a high level of circulating parathyroid hormone occurs in response to a chronically lowered plasma calcium. The causes may be:

(1) Vitamin D deficiency from poor dietary intake, lack of ultraviolet light, steatorrhoea or post-surgery of the small bowel,

(2) Renal failure, which is the commonest cause of secondary hyperparathyroidism due to a failure of formation of the active form of vitamin D.

The serum calcium is low to normal in secondary hyperparathyroidism and the diagnosis is made on the basis of radiological changes of hyperparathyroidism plus a raised serum parathormone level.

TERTIARY HYPERPARATHYROIDISM

What is it?

This is a term given to autonomous secretion of parathyroid hormone irrespective of the ionized calcium level. It occurs in people who have secondary hyperparathyroidism of long standing, presumably by development of an adenoma in previously hyperplastic parathyroid glands. When hypercalcaemia develops under these circumstances tertiary hyperparathyroidism is probably present.

HYPOFUNCTION OF THE PARATHYROIDS

What is it?

This occurs when there is a diminished secretion of PTH. The most common cause is following disruption to the blood supply or inadvertent removal of the glands during thyroid surgery. Other causes of hypoparathyroidism are congenital absence of the glands (a condition usually seen in children and very rare) and autoimmune destruction of the glands. All causes of hypoparathyroidism are rare.

Pseudohypoparathyroidism

What is it?

This is a sex-linked dominantly inherited disease and is associated with characteristic abnormalities of appearance and physical and mental retardation, and is thought to be due to a failure of the end organ to respond to PTH, resulting in hypocalcaemia and hyperphosphataemia.

Clinical features of hypoparathyroidism

Mostly these are the features of tetany. They are due to low concentration of calcium in the extracellular fluid and consist of numbness and tingling of the fingers and around the lips, carpopedal spasm and occasionally laryngeal stridor. Convulsions, abdominal pain and vomiting and epileptic fits all occur. Hypocalcaemic tetany can be confirmed in mild cases by Trousseau's sign, that is by producing limb ischaemia with a sphygmomanometer cuff inflated above systolic pressure for 2 minutes. Carpopedal spasm occurs during the course of the test. Psychiatric change such as depression is very common in hypocalcaemia. A few people, particularly with juvenile onset, will develop cataracts and abnormalities of the nails and teeth.

Assessment and investigations

The plasma calcium level is low, the plasma inorganic phosphate level is raised and the plasma alkaline phosphatase level is normal.

Contrast the findings in osteomalacia where plasma calcium and phosphate levels are both low and alkaline phosphatase is raised.

In pseudohypoparathyroidism the serum parathormone level is greatly elevated.

X-ray changes

In longstanding hypoparathyroidism calcification of the basal ganglia occurs. In pseudohypoparathyroidism there are characteristic skeletal anomalies including short metacarpal bones.

Management

Treatment can be given by way of vitamin D analogues in large dosage. Usually 0.5–2.0 mg per day of calciferol is required.

After care

These patients need lifelong follow-up with close monitoring of serum calcium levels.

HOW TO MEASURE THE SERUM CALCIUM – HOW ACCURATELY IN GENERAL PRACTICE

Spurious results often occur due to inappropriate collection of blood. 10 ml of blood should be taken from a fasting patient using a non-occluded vein and sent as soon as possible to the laboratory. Repeat tests are usually required to establish whether hypercalcaemia truly exists.

SUMMARY OF PARATHYROID GLAND DISORDERS

Disorders of the parathyroid gland are extremely rare and unlikely to be discovered except biochemically in general practice. However, a working knowledge of calcium metabolism is important as rickets still occurs in isolated Asian communities in this country. It is important to be able to recognize the symptoms of hypercalcaemia which may require urgent hospital admission to treat the immediate condition and look for the underlying cause.

Case history

Case history of a white male, with multiple endocrine abnormalities

First attended aged 43 with a 4 year history of vomiting and abdominal pain. Known heavy drinker. Large duodenal ulcer found on endoscopy. Underwent vagotomy and pyloroplasty. Following year (1972) an emergency laparotomy for perforation of stoma. Given Polya gastrectomy. Same year passed renal stone. Apparently normal calcium.

Aged 47 (1976) acute haematemesis – chronic stomal ulceration. Serum gastrin levels grossly elevated. *Zollinger–Ellison* syndrome diagnosed. Total gastrectomy performed. Normal pancreas observed.

1976. Developed left sided chest pains. Normal e.c.g. No diagnosis.

1977. Haemoglobin 6.49 g/100 ml, macrocytic anaemia presumed secondary to gastrectomy. Started B_{12} injections.

1980. Further chest pains.

1982. Alcohol problems exacerbated. Routine LFTs unmasked raised calcium and low phosphate. Ca 2.98, P 0.55, Alk. Phos. 218.

Hyperparathyroidism suspected. Further biochemical evaluations revealed low plasma Vit. D and urinary hydroxyproline. Bone scan revealed healing pathological fractures in ribs – pituitary fossa was normal.

After considerable difficulty a thallium scan isolated a parathyroid adenoma which was subsequently removed, after which his calcuim returned to normal.

He continues to drink heavily.

OSTEOPOROSIS

What is it?

Osteoporosis is a common bone disease causing pain and disability particularly in the elderly. In osteoporosis the total mass of bone is reduced, and there is less bone tissue per unit volume of 'bone' but the composition of the bone tissue in terms of the balance of mineral and organic components is normal. There are a number of causes and it is difficult to draw the line between 'normal' bone loss with age and the onset of osteoporosis. This is particularly true of women where some degree of postmenopausal osteoporosis is ubiquitous. Only a few women, however, develop clinical features. Other causes of osteoporosis are:

(1)   Cushing's syndrome (or exogenous steroid therapy)
(2)   hypogonadism
(3)   immobilization

Clinical features

Bone pain is common, particularly in the back. Fractures occur in the vertebrae, femoral necks and wrist. Generally vertebral fractures occur at intervals with a sudden onset, severe back pain for 1 or 2 months and then resolution. Loss of height occurs.

Assessment and investigations

Plasma calcium phosphate and alkaline phosphatase levels are normal. Radiology shows loss of bone density though this is very insensitive. Crush fractures of the vertebrae are common.

Management

In postmenopausal osteoporosis up to the age of 70, treatment with oestrogen (balanced with a progestogen to reduce the risk of uterine carcinoma) will retard the rate of bone loss. There is no other specific treatment for osteoporosis. Avoid immobilization as much as possible and treat pain.

PAGET'S DISEASE OF BONE

What is it?

Paget's disease is a localized disease of bone, which may affect only one bone or any bone in the body. The cause is unknown, although the recent discovery of inclusion bodies in osteoclasts suggests a slow virus may be responsible. It is characterized by increased bone resorption locally with secondary bone formation and sclerosis. The newly modelled bone is abnormal and pathologically weak. It also has an increased blood flow. Paget's disease is very common in the middle aged and elderly of both sexes.

Clinical features

Most people suffering from Paget's disease are asymptomatic. In about 10% of patients the following occur:

(1)   bone pain,
(2)   deformity,
(3)   pathological fracture,
(4)   nerve compression syndromes (including deafness),
(5)   high output cardiac failure,
(6)   osteosarcomatous change (less than 1%).

Assessment and investigations

Plasma calcium and phosphate levels are normal except in immobilization, when hypercalcaemia may occur. Plasma alkaline phosphatase levels are extremely high.

Radiological changes are characteristic. Localized areas of radio-translucency caused by bone resorption occur (resorption fronts, osteoporosis circumscripta). Later cycles of bone resorption with secondary bone formation occur leaving a coarse abnormal trabecular pattern with mixed sclerosis and rarefaction in an expanded bone.

Management

Most symptomatic patients can be managed with analgesics. Calcitonin which inhibits bone resorption is used in selected cases only with the advice of the endocrinologist. Didronal may also be used.

5
ENDOCRINE DISEASES OF THE OVARY AND BREAST

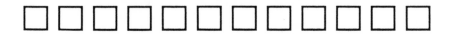

WHAT ARE THEY?

The ovaries are the female gonads. As with other endocrine organs we can categorize ovarian endocrine disorders broadly as hypofunction and hyperfunction though this is not completely satisfactory. We shall consider the following clinical entities:

(1) Hypogonadism in the female: a state characterized by inadequate supply of gonadal steroid hormones to the tissues;

(2) Puberty problems in the female;

(3) Assessment of ovarian function in infertility problems;

(4) Hirsutism and virilization: hirsutism is 'inappropriate' hairiness in a female; virilization is the development of more serious features of androgenization;

(5) Disorders of sex differentiation;

(6) Endocrinologically active tumours of the ovary;

(7) Endocrine disorders of the breast.

Table 9 Laboratory findings in endocrine disorders affecting ovarian function

Condition	Serum hormone estimation						Comments
	LH	FSH	Oestrodiol	Prolactin	Testosterone	17-Hydroxy-progesterone	
Ovarian failure	↑	↑	↓	N	N	N	Absent or diseased ovaries
Hyperprolactin-aemia	N	N	N/↓	↑	N	N	Usually 'post pill'; with pituitary adenoma; or no cause found
Hypopituitarism other than with high prolactin including anorexia nervosa	↓	↓	↓	N/↓	N/↓	N	Other hypopituitary signs; X-ray the skull
Polycystic ovaries	↑ or N	N	N	N	N/↑	N	High LH/FSH ratio; obese, hirsute; ovaries enlarged
Ovarian masculinizing tumour	N	N	N	N	↑	N	Evidence of virilization; ovarian mass
Ovarian oestrogen secreting tumour	↓	N/↓	↑	N	N	N	Irregular menses; ovarian mass
Adrenal source of androgens: Cushing's	N	N	N	N	↑	↑	Looks Cushingoid; do serum cortisol
tumour	N	N	N	N	↑	↑	Virilized; do urinary steroids
adrenogenital syndrome	N	N	N	N	N/↑	↑	Virilized; can be partial
Normal values	3.0–12 (P) 25–64 (O) 2.4–13 (L)	0.5 – 5.0 u/l	74–368 (P) 735–1840(O) 368–1100(L)	<600 iu/l	< 2.5 nmol/l	< 12 nmol/l	

P = proliferative phase, O = ovulatory values, L = luteal phase of normal menstrual cycle

94

WHAT PROBLEMS?

The most troublesome problems are as follows:

(1) A major problem is that all the above conditions cut across the usual specialty basis of hospital practice. There is an as-yet undeveloped role for the GP in helping to coordinate these specialist services and in follow-up. The liaison does not always work entirely smoothly at present despite the development of combined specialist clinics.

(2) Some of the disorders mentioned are extremely prevalent – particularly in general practice.

(3) Some, in particular hirsutism and infertility, are still resistant to therapy despite recent advances.

(4) There is a very large amount of stress and psychological suffering in relation to these disorders (which are so relevant to sexuality) that is not managed particularly well under existing circumstances.

(5) One of the problems facing the general practitioner interested in this area is access to and interpretation of the appropriate investigations (see Table 9).

(6) The most important problem is that these disorders are embarrassing and threatening to a great number of patients and doctors and require sympathetic handling. Often however the problems remain submerged and so inaccessible to the most careful handling.

HYPOGONADISM IN THE FEMALE

Aetiology

It is useful to consider two groups: (1) failure of normal development and (2) failure of established sexual development.

These two groups are often referred to as primary and secondary amenorrhoea, this being an obvious clinical feature, though amenorrhoea does not always mean hypogonadism is present (see Table 10).

Table 10   Hypogonadism/amenorrhoea

Primary amenorrhoea	Secondary amenorrhoea
Congenital absence of ovaries (several syndromes)	Not seen with absent ovaries but is with hypoplastic ovaries.
Acquired disease of the ovary (any cause)	Otherwise any cause of 1° amenorrhoea though with different likelihoods of occurrence
Hypopituitarism (any cause)	Pregnancy. Oral contraceptives (amenorrhoea but not hypogonadism)
Androgenization (any cause)	Hyperprolactinaemic states

The illustration is designed to be easy to remember rather than to be totally comprehensive. It does not include anatomical abnormalities such as absent uterus or imperforate hymen nor does it include testicular feminization

Further details

Congenital absence

(1)   Turner's syndrome
(2)   Pure ovarian agenesis

Acquired disease

(1)   Surgical removal
(2)   Radiation
(3)   Mumps
(4)   Granulomatous and neoplastic replacement

Hypopituitarism

(1) 'Functional' hypothalamopituitary disease. Low gonadotrophins with low oestrogen levels in serum. A failure of normal feedback mechanisms.
(2) Organic pituitary disease such as pituitary tumour.
(3) Hyperprolactinaemic states cause hypogonadism by impairing pituitary gonadotrophin release and by an ovarian mechanism.
(4) Anorexia nervosa, *any condition* causing severe weight loss or catabolism. Also obesity.

Androgenization

(1) Ovarian tumours
(2) Polycystic ovarian syndrome (also with obesity)
(3) Cushing's syndrome
(4) Congenital adrenal hyperplasia
(5) Adrenal tumours

Clinical features

Hypogonadism usually presents as amenorrhoea or oligomenorrhoea. Other features:

(1) lack of sexual libido
(2) dyspareunia from small or dry vagina
(3) breast atrophy

which are all due to oestrogen lack, can be elicited often but are not usually presenting features.

When the presentation is primary amenorrhoea, the person's problem is usually delayed or absent puberty and this will be considered later in this chapter. When the presentation is secondary amenorrhoea the person's problem may be infertility, sexual difficulties or most frequently, anxiety about not being 'normal'.

Assessment and investigation

The genital organs must be examined in all cases of amenorrhoea but:

(1) Only if the examiner is competent to assess all the findings,
(2) On the minimum number of occasions that will provide definitive results, and
(3) By an appropriate method.

For instance, in a young girl with primary amenorrhoea one examination under anaesthetic, perhaps with laparoscopy and ovarian biopsy, could replace several distressing examinations.

Assessment of primary amenorrhoea will be considered in the section on puberty problems.

Assessment of secondary amenorrhoea

When a woman presents with secondary amenorrhoea assess the case as follows.

(1) Could she be pregnant? Examine and test.

(2) Was gonadal function previously normal? What was the age of menarche and the frequency of menstruation prior to the amenorrhoea and when did it start?

(3) Has there been recent psychological stress, fear of pregnancy etc?

(4) Has there been marked weight loss (or weight gain)? This probably operates via hypopituitarism.

(5) Is there evidence of severe or chronic extragenital disease? This probably operates via hypopituitarism.

(6) Any history of disease that could affect the ovaries: surgery near them; radiation; mumps; chronic tuberculosis or sarcoid or amyloid, iron deposition diseases, autoimmune disease of thyroid or adrenal, endometriosis?

(7) Is there evidence of androgenization?: hirsutism, increasing muscularity; voice changes; clitoromegaly; ovarian mass; Cushing's syndrome.

(8) Is she on 'the pill' or was she on it prior to the amenorrhoea developing?

(9) Is she on any other relevant drugs such as androgens, anabolic steroids?

(10) Is there galactorrhoea? Examine the breasts. (Usually 'post-pill' or with a pituitary adenoma or no cause found.)

(11) Is there evidence of a pituitary cause? Galactorrhoea; examine for loss of pubic and axillary hair; hypothyroidism; pale fine skin of hypopituitarism; headache; bitemporal visual field loss; skull X-ray for pituitary tumour.

Causal groupings

Such an assessment will cover the main causal groupings:

(1) inadequate ovarian function from birth,
(2) ovarian damage subsequently,
(3) hypopituitarism (remember that hyperprolactinaemia causes hypopituitarism by suppressing normal output of gonadotrophic hormones), and
(4) abnormal androgens from ovary adrenal or exogenous sources.

Special investigations

Following are the appropriate special investigations that are available. They are not all needed in every case.

(1) An adequate pelvic assessment to exclude ovarian masses and anatomical abnormalities (essential);
(2) Ovarian ultrasound examination for ovarian masses and polycystic ovaries;

(3)   Laparosocopy and ovarian biopsy;

(4)   Laparotomy when ovarian tumour is strongly suspected;

(5)   Pituitary fossa tomography for assessment of the pituitary fossa;

(6)   Computer assisted tomographic (CAT) scans with contrast enhancement for assessment of the pituitary fossa;

(7)   CAT scans of adrenal and other adrenal imaging techniques.

Management

Specific

Ovarian failure

This requires replacement therapy with oestrogens and proges-togens to encourage breast development and vaginal maturation. The simplest regime is to use a 30 μg oestrogen contraceptive pill cyclically. Oestrogens are dangerous drugs and higher doses should be used with caution. Osteoporosis may occur in later life unless ovarian failure is treated.

Polycystic ovaries (PCO)

A weight reduction regimen is the foremost need. If hirsutism is prominent this should be specifically treated (*see below)* if desired. Infertility with PCO is not usually a problem after diagnosis since ovulation can usually be induced with clomiphene 50 mg a day for 5 days, starting again after the ensuing menstrual bleeding ceases. Oral contraceptives are *usually* contraindicated for fear of sup-pressing the pituitary ovarian axis.

Hyperprolactinaemia

Stop the contraceptive pill, and assess the pituitary fossa carefully with tomography and if necessary CAT scanning. A definite pituit-ary adenoma may require surgery, usually by the transsphenoidal route. Hyperprolactinaemia usually responds to the dopamine agonist bromocriptine. Start 2.5 mg *nocte* and increase by 2.5 mg after food every 48 hours until the serum prolactin is controlled. Usually 5–10 mg a day is enough. Side-effects are prominent – nausea, vomiting, hypotension and Raynaud's phenomenon. Continue long term with monitoring of serum prolactin and pituitary fossa X-rays when used for pituitary tumours – usually for 6 months in 'post-pill' amenorrhoea/galactorrhoea. Pituitary tumours should be followed-up in a specialist clinic though the GP can also be involved. Do not re-start the person on oral contraceptives.

'Functional' hypothalamopituitary failure

This is a low gonadotrophic state with low levels of gonadal steroids – a failure of feedback mechanisms without evidence of organic pituitary disease or hyperprolactinaemia. Once this has been identified:

(1)   Oral contraceptives are totally contra-indicated,

(2)   Clomiphene cyclically to induce ovulation and re-start 'cycling' can be tried,

(3)   If clomiphene in maximum dosage (200 mg per day for 5 days cyclically approached gradually) fails, then assessment of the ovary to establish the presence of normal follicles is necessary before considering exogenous gonadotroph therapy,

(4)   Exogenous gonadotroph therapy with FSH and HCG is given in specialized clinics to induce ovulation. This should never be attempted by the GP.

Organic hypopituitarism

See Chapter 7, on Pituitary Disease, for specific therapy.

Oestrogen and progestogen therapy with cyclical oral contraceptive is usually required.

101

Anorexia nervosa and variants

The specific treatment is to achieve weight gain by specialized management techniques.

Never give the contraceptive pill.

Ovarian tumours

Surgical assessment is mandatory.

Cushing's, adrenal tumours, adrenogenital syndrome

For treatment of these conditions, see Chapter 8, on the Adrenal Glands.

Symptomatic treatment

Amenorrhoea should never be treated symptomatically. It may be treated expectantly on occasions. Anxieties can be explored and areas of stress identified. Remember that even oligomenorrhoea may mean anovulatory cycles and a serious suppression of the pituitary–ovarian axis that could be rendered permanent by inappropriate oestrogen administration.

Information for patient and family

Factors always to be borne in mind are as follows:

(1) The weight – over- and underweight states radically affect gonadal function.

(2) The place of stress.

(3) Sexuality. Very often anxieties about interpersonal relations, ageing and femininity are presented as concern 'with the periods' or excessive hairiness or dyspareunia.

(4) Fertility. The implications for present and future fertility of 'the diagnosis' should always be made clear to a woman.

(5) Dangers of oestrogen therapy (*see below*) must be balanced against the benefits of therapy and the risks of not giving it.

(6) Particular care should be taken when chromosomal and ovarian disease is present. The idea that she is 'not a woman', once implanted, can destroy not only a marriage but a whole personality.

There is a most important role for the GP in the area of personal intimate advice.

Prevention

Once again, inappropriate prescription of the contraceptive pill for menstrual irregularity cannot be too strongly condemned. Timely advice to teenage girls who embark on radical weight reduction programmes can prevent hypogonadism supervening. Similarly, advice to the obese can help.

PUBERTY

What is it?

Puberty refers to the onset of secondary sexual characteristics following normal activation of the gonad by pituitary gonadotrophic hormone. Here we deal with delayed puberty including the assessment of primary amenorrhoea and precocious puberty. In Britain today, normal puberty in girls has fairly wide limits of onset between 9 and 13 years. Precocious puberty may be said to be present when secondary sexual characteristics appear before this time. Delayed puberty may be said to be present when secondary sexual characteristics have not appeared by the end of this time. Constitutional delay in growth and adolescence is only present provided there is no other cause present (as detailed in the previous section). The average age of menarche in Britain is 13 with a normal range of 11 – 15. These same observations also apply to boys and although the onset of puberty in boys is a little later it is not as much as is generally considered to be the case, because the onset of pubertal changes in the male is not so easily recognizable and 10 – 15 are reasonable limits.

(1)   These wide limits can be used to reassure families.
(2)   Nevertheless it is possible to identify 'delay' or abnormality within the age limits.

The assessment of primary amenorrhoea is in reality often the assessment of puberty.

What problems

The most pressing problem is anxiety in the person affected and the parent. Most people referred for investigation of delayed puberty, and precocious puberty, have neither and are perfectly normal people. The belief of the public is that normal puberty occurs within much narrower age limits than is actually the case. Nevertheless severe psychological problems (usually in boys but also in girls) can occur when adolescents drop behind their sibs and schoolmates in the development race. Knowledge of how to grade pubertal development needs to be widely disseminated among doctors because of the relevance of this topic to general practice.

Other problems are:

(1)   short stature
(2)   tall stature
(3)   precocious puberty.

Clinical features

The clinical features of delayed puberty are lack of normal secondary sexual characteristics.

In the female, puberty can be graded by reference to breast development (B), graded from 1 to 5. Bl is prepubertal and B5 is adult.

In both sexes, gradation can be made by reference to pubic hair development (PH), grades 1 to 5. PH1 is nil and PH5 is adult – although development of the male escutcheon is still later (6).

In the male the genital development (G) replaces that of the breast: 1 is prepubertal and 5 is mature. Enlargement of the testis is the primary event in the pubertal development of the male genitalia.

Short stature is usually associated with delayed puberty and tall stature with precocious puberty but this is not always the case.

Presence of pubic and axillary hair in girls without breast development may indicate an abnormal source of androgens, as does penile enlargement without testicular enlargement in boys.

Assessment and investigations

Basically assessment answers the following questions:

(1) Is the girl in fact normal?
(2) Is this a problem of constitutional delay in growth and adolescence with no serious illness?
(3) Is there some other disturbance present, as designated in the section on hypogonadism?
(4) Is there some other cause of short or tall stature?
(5) Is precocious puberty present and if so is it constitutional or is there some other cause?

Normality can often be established if pubertal changes have in fact begun and it can be expected if the girl is well within the normal age limits for puberty or if there is a family history of 'delayed' puberty or precocious puberty. Always measure the height and weight of the girl and enter these on the centile charts. Assess the degree of pubertal development and the 'expected' range of the girl's adult height by reference to the heights of the biological parents. Similarly take note of the mother's and father's age of puberty.

Look for evidence of other diseases as indicated under the following headings.

(1) Chronic debilitating illness: asthma, renal failure, heart disease, cystic fibrosis, Crohn's disease, coeliac disease – *short stature* will be present.

(2) Hypopituitarism: clinical features referrable to lack of thyroid adrenal and growth hormones – *short stature* will be present.

(3) Ovarian absence or disease: features of Turner's syndrome (short stature, web neck, breast absence, wide carrying angle) or eunuchoidism (long arms and legs for the body height).

(4) Androgenization: pubic and axillary hair but no breast development. One cause is congenital adrenal hyperplasia.

(5) Hypothalamic: brain damage or tumour from many causes can cause both delayed and precocious puberty. Ask about epilepsy, meningitis, encephalitis.

   In addition if tall stature is the problem think of Marfan's syndrome and homocystinuria.

(6) In precocious puberty precocious adrenarche may occur normally 1–2 years in advance of pubertal development.

(7) It is usually constitutional with or without tall stature or obesity.

(8) It may be hypothalamic with brain tumour (commoner in boys), brain damage or polyostotic fibrous dysplasia.

(9) It can be due to ovarian (or testicular) tumour.

(10) Beware adrenal hyperplasia (or tumour that can stimulate it).

In assessing any adolescent with a pubertal problem try to link together the chronological age, expected age for the height, expected age for the degree of pubertal development and expected age for the degree of somatic development shown on bone age. The odd one out will often become apparent in this way. At the same time link the state of affairs to the young person's social and psychological background and the biological background in terms of parental characteristics. Remember that puberty is a graded and orderly phenomenon so that considerable pubic hair development without breast development is likely to be abnormal, as is penile enlargement without prior testicular enlargement.

Investigations which are helpful include:

(1) Stage the pubertal development accurately;

(2) Bone age by X-ray of the wrist:

   (a) it may be advanced in abnormal androgenization or where the problem is, say, an imperforate hymen causing amenorrhoea

   (b) it will be delayed in hypopituitarism and gonadal disease but may not be appropriate to the height or the degree of pubertal development

   (c) in constitutional delay in growth and adolescence the girl's height, somatic development (bone age) and pubertal development will all come together for a child of less chronological age;

(3) X-ray of the pituitary fossa;

(4) Chromosome analysis. Turner's syndrome is 45, X;

(5) Pelvic assessment by a gynaecologist is essential and this may include laparoscopy and ovarian biopsy;

(6) Serum FSH and LH levels in serum: these hormone estimations will be high in all forms of ovarian failure but will be low in constitutional delay in growth and adolescence and pituitary failure;

(7) Serum oestrodiol (or in boys serum testosterone);

(8)   Serum prolactin in pituitary and hypothalamic disease;

(9)   LHRH test: absent response in pituitary disease, sluggish in hypothalamic disease. Exaggerated response with elevated basal levels of LH and FSH in hypothalamic precocious puberty;

(10)   HCG test in boys to determine testicular responsiveness;

(11)   Serum 17-hydroxyprogesterone level to exclude congenital adrenal hyperplasia in precocious puberty;

(12)   CAT scan where neurological or pituitary disease is suspected.

Management of specific conditions

Guidelines are as follows.

(1)   Any serious disease should be treated as far as possible.

(2)   Management of hypopituitary disease and abnormal androgenization : this will be considered in later sections.

(3)   Ovarian failure should be managed by cyclical treatment with a 30 μg oestrogen contraceptive pill. This will induce breast development and if a uterus is present encourage monthly withdrawal bleeding.

(4)   Management of infertility: this will be considered in a later section.

(5)   In constitutional delay in growth and adolescence it is sometimes necessary to institute treatment because of anxiety or psychological trauma. This is rarely necessary in girls (unless there is some organic dysfunction) since the social pressure upon them is less. In boys treatment with HCG can be given.

(6)   Tall stature may be due to constitutional factors. Usually the parents request treatment for a girl.

Treatment with oestrogen/progestogen replacement as above can be given to hasten closure of the epiphyses but is recommended only when the expected adult height is greater than 6 feet (1.8 metres).

(7) Precocious puberty:
    (a) If constitutional and not severe no specific treatment is given,
    (b) If constitutional but severe (more than 3 years' advance) then bone age advance can be slowed with cyproterone acetate, an antiandrogen, in girls or boys, or medroxyprogesterone acetate works well in girls,
    (c) If a tumour or other serious condition is present it should be treated on its merits.

Symptomatic treatment

Considerable reassurance is needed for both the adolescents involved and their parents.

Information to person involved and family

It is helpful to demonstrate the growth and development charts to the family as an aid to explanation and a demonstration that future events can be predicted on a scientific basis.

The link to the parents' own puberty is often very helpful in allaying anxiety.

Often early signs of puberty are present and have not been noticed and this can be reassuring.

Perfectly normal development is to be expected in cases of constitutional delay and this should be emphasized.

Fantasies such as 'I'm changing sex' (common with gynaecomastia), 'I'll never grow up' or 'I'll always be small' are often present and should be opened up for discussion.

Prevention

Prevention of puberty problems is not possible.

Aftercare

(1) Anyone who is taking hormone therapy requires careful long term monitoring preferably by the GP after stabilization of therapy.

(2) A balance should be struck in adolescents with delayed puberty – too much investigation or hospital visiting can convince them that they are sexually abnormal. Provided proper assessment is undertaken initially and serious disease excluded, follow-up is best undertaken by the GP.

(3) Once reasonable pubertal development has occurred the adolescent should no longer be followed-up.

INFERTILITY

What is it?

Infertility is the problem of a couple, *not* a person. It can be considered present when no pregnancy results from regular (2 – 3 times per week) unguarded intercourse for 1 year.

What problems?

(1) It is essential that both partners are involved in infertility assessments from the start, since it is common to find more than one contributing factor. Usually only one partner (the woman) presents but this should be gently discouraged and both partners seen and investigated together. This minimizes the 'his fault – her fault' attitude.

(2) Men are by and large reluctant to have infertility investigation and may need sympathetic handling.

(3) Infertility assessments require the skills of more than one medical attendant. Liaison between gynaecologist, endocrine physician, urologist and general practitioner is often far from perfect.

Clinical features

Causes of infertility are summarized in Table 11.

Table 11   Causes of infertility

In the male	In the female
Testicular disease	*Ovarian disease*
– Klinefelter's	– Turner's
– undescended or late	– hypoplasia
descended testis	– radiation or removal
– mumps, orchitis	– mumps, oophoritis
Hypopituitarism	*Hypopituitarism*
– panhypopituitarism	
– isolated hypogonadotrophic	
hypogonadism	
Mechanical	*Mechanical*
– absent vas	– blocked fallopian tubes
– epididymo-orchitis	– other anatomical abnormalities
– prostatitis	
Suppressed testis	*Suppressed ovaries*
– androgen therapy	– oestrogen therapy
– antimitotic agents	

Attributable to both partners
Failure of normal sexual relations through low frequency of intercourse, partial or inadequate intercourse, impotence and frigidity

The woman

(1) There may be hypogonadism as previously described, features of hypopituitarism or androgenization.

(2) A search for galactorrhoea is essential.

(3) A detailed menstrual history is essential as even minor irregularities of the cycle may indicate anovulatory menses.

(4) Complete gynaecological assessment is necessary.

(5) Note any abnormal weight loss or gain.

The man

(1) Evidence of hypogonadism or hypopituitarism should be sought.

(2) The size of the testes is directly related to seminiferous tubular mass and so small testes are a good indicator of damage and a reduced capacity to produce sperm. Normally-sized testes do not, however, mean the sperm count is normal.

(3) Ensure both testes are normally present and there is no history of late descent or maldescent, no hernia operations particularly in childhood.

(4) Examine (standing the man upright) for varicocoeles.

(5) Ask for a history of mumps orchitis or trauma.

(6) In Klinefelter's syndrome the testes are quite characteristically firm and very small (pea-sized to nil).

In both

Enquire (separately) for venereal disease.

Assessment and investigations

First decide in consultation with the couple when and if investigations should commence – depending on age, children by previous marriages and other factors. Normally both partners should be investigated simultaneously and seen as a couple whenever possible.

In the woman

Confirmation of ovulation should be obtained. Instruction in keeping a basal body temperature chart and documentation of the cycle is essential. A serum progesterone done during the luteal phase will confirm ovulation in that cycle. If there is any suspicion on menstrual history or temperature chart that ovulation is not occurring, then a serum oestrodiol prolactin and LH and FSH levels should be obtained (*see* Table 9).

Provided the partner is not azoospermic, the woman should next have tests of tubal patency and, if ovarian disease or pelvic pathology is suspected, laparoscopy and ovarian biopsy.

In the man

The man should have at least two seminal specimens analysed.

(1)   Specimens should be complete not partial.
(2)   The man should not have an intercurrent illness or have had a recent intercurrent illness.

In both

A sexual history should be obtained and an estimate made of the couple's mutual concern and attachment. Infertility investigations can be protracted and can cause or exacerbate marital disharmony.

Investigations

Endocrine investigations should be interpreted as previously detailed.

Seminal analysis

A sperm density of greater than 20 million per ml is probably normal. Motility is probably more important than density. Low motility may indicate the presence of sperm antibodies in the man. Sperm antibodies in the woman's serum are another cause of infertility. A low volume may indicate an incomplete specimen (with loss of the sperm-rich fraction) or too frequent ejaculations.

Note the presence of pus cells and culture for organisms if present.

Management of specific problems

Anovulation

(1) Ovarian failure (high FSH and LH levels) cannot be treated.

(2) Organic pituitary disease can be treated by induction of ovulation with gonadotrophins.

(3) 'Functional' anovulatory states are treated with clomiphene 50 mg a day for 5 days. Ovulation should occur at around the tenth day after commencing therapy. The dose can be increased stepwise to 200 mg a day for 5 days. Failure to respond can be treated with gonadotrophins provided the ovary is normal. This is done by daily injections of human menopausal gonadotroph until oestrogen levels rise to satisfactory. Then ovulation is induced by a single injection of HCG. This should never be attempted without full hospital cover. HCG can cause nausea and vomiting.

(4) Hyperprolactinaemia (with or without galactorrhoea) suppresses ovulation. It can be treated with bromocriptine starting with 2.5 mg nocte. Hyperprolactinaemia also causes male infertility.

114

Mechanical problems

Blocked fallopian tubes or ligated vasa can be operated upon. The success rate is about one in five for subsequent pregnancy.

Sperm antibodies

In the male, steroids can be tried.

In the female, use of a condom for 6 months may allow levels to decline.

Low sperm density

There are many suggested remedies but in general very little can be done. Never give systemic androgen therapy as this depresses sperm production.

Varicocoele

If the varicocoele is large, surgical treatment (to the internal spermatic plexus, not on the varicocoele itself) is justified. It elevates the sperm density but has less effect on conception rates.

Symptomatic treatment

Constant attention to the couple's state of mind and to their tolerance of investigations that pinpoint their 'differentness' and 'inferior' status is necessary.

Information to patient and family

(1)   Up to 20% of couples are infertile.

(2)   Fertility is the facility of a couple. Women are not 'barren' and virility and fertility are quite separate in men.

(3)   Advice as to adoption procedures.

Prevention

Immunization could prevent mumps orchitis in men.

Correct (early) identification and treatment of undescended testicles is of the utmost importance.

Do not give oestrogens without investigation to women with oligomenorrhoea.

After care

Fertility and infertility are closely allied to sexuality and there is a large scope for continued support for couples with problems in this field.

HIRSUTISM AND VIRILISM

What are they?

Hirsutism refers to the presence of excess facial and or body hair in women. Virilism refers to the development of other signs of androgenization in addition to hirsutism (Table 12).

Clinical features

The clinical features of hirsutism are dealt with below, under Assessment. Certain sites for hair growth are more characteristically 'male':

(1)   upper lip and chin,
(2)   nose and ears,

Table 12 Causes of hirsutism and virilism

Causes of hirsutism and virilization	Comment	Details
Constitutional hirsutism: no abnormal source of androgens	Includes familial, racial, normal ageing and sexuality fears	Menses normal. No biochemical abnormalities. Probably receptor sensitivity. No virilization
Ovarian source of abnormal androgens	Polycystic ovary. Masculinizing tumour of the ovary	Menses usually affected Virilization may be present
Adrenal source of abnormal androgens	Congenital adrenal hyperplasia Adrenal carcinoma Cushing's syndrome	Menses affected Virilization present
Exogenous source of androgens	Drug history	Menses probably affected Virilization my be present

(3) fingers and toes,
(4) upper abdomen and
(5) chest and back.

In addition women with polycystic ovaries may be obese.

Similarly evidence of virilism is most important. Such signs include:

(1) loss or irregularity of the periods,
(2) voice deepening and thyroid cartilage protrusion,
(3) clitoral hypertrophy,
(4) atrophy of the breasts,
(5) temporal recession of the hairline and
(6) increased muscle bulk with broad shoulders, muscular arms and narrowed hips (the male bodily habitus).

What problems?

(1) The definition of what is a normal degree of hairiness is difficult. Many women complain of 'hairiness' when they have a problem with a relationship or fear that they are getting older or losing their femininity. This is therefore really a problem concerning sexuality and should be recognized as such.

(2) A further factor is that our society encourages women to a self-image of a 'glamour girl type' which is just plainly not the reality of the situation. The range of normal is in fact much wider than some have been led to believe.

(3) This is not to say that serious psychological upset cannot be caused by a degree of hairiness which is medically 'normal' – It can.

(4) What it does mean is that the medical effort should not be on endocrine investigations in such a woman but on the more appropriate support – psychotherapy and cosmetic lines.

(5)   The additional fact that hirsutism is extremely difficult to treat means that, even in women with 'excessive' hair by anyone's standards, these factors assume probably the greatest significance in the management of hirsutism.

Assessment

The first decision is whether the hirsutism lies within the range of normal after giving consideration to the following matters.

(1)   The family history – does the mother have a problem (or have the sisters).

(2)   The racial background – mediterranean and middle-eastern races have more hair than nordic types. In addition, of course black hair always looks more noticeable. Enquire as to parents' and grandparents' origins.

(3)   The age of the woman – older women normally get more hairy.

(4)   The extent of the hirsutism – it is normal (taking account of item (5), below) to have a few hairs on the chin, a light moustache, a few hairs on the nipples, a male escutcheon or hair on the medial upper thighs. Similarly hairiness of the forearms and backs of thighs and certainly the lower legs is often seen.

(5)   Crucial to the decision is the length of time the hair has been present. In constitutional hirsutism the problem usually begins at puberty. In tumour of the ovary or adrenal the history is usually short. A useful question is to ask if hair appeared on a new area of the body – since it is difficult to distinguish a slow history of the hairiness 'getting worse' from static hairiness with increased anxiety about it.

(6)   Disturbance of the menstrual cycle. This is crucial, since most women with constitutional hirsutism will have regular periods and most women with a serious organic pathology will lose their periods.

119

(7)   Features of virilism confirm a serious pathology.

(8)   Take a drug history – anabolic steroids, testosterone (for the menopause), progestogens in contraceptive pills and phenytoin for epilepsy can all induce hirsutism.

Investigations

These should be requested only when the doctor has made the decision that significant hirsutism exists – not in every case. If in doubt, referral is appropriate. Investigations are not only expensive but frequently not productive. They can also be time consuming for the woman. Features of virilization always require investigation.

(1)   Request:
    (a)   serum testosterone
    (b)   serum 17-hydroxyprogesterone (17-OHP)
    (c)   androstenedione
    (d)   dehydroepiandosterone (DHEA); and sulphate DHEAS

(2)   Do not request:
    (e)   24 hour urinary 17-oxo and 17-oxogenic steroids

In constitutional hirsutism all tests are normal.

In PCO a normal or slightly raised testosterone is found.

In masculinizing ovarian tumour a high testosterone is found.

A raised 17-OHP suggests adrenogenital syndrome.

Elevated androstenedione points to an ovarian rather than adrenal overproduction of androgens and DHEA the reverse.

In addition, if Cushing's syndrome is suspected tests for that are appropriate.

Occasionally dynamic tests are helpful in indicating treatment regimes:

(1)   androgens may be suppressed by dexamethasone
(2)   androgens may be suppressed by oestrogen therapy

If an ovarian tumour is suspected then laparoscopy of laparotomy may be needed. Sometimes it has been found necessary to split the ovary to locate a small tumour. Adrenal tumours are located by appropriate adrenal imaging techniques including intravenous urography (i.v.u.) aortography with selective catheterization and CAT scans.

Management

Specific

The following regimes are available.

(1)   Ovarian masculinizing tumour – surgical removal;

(2)   Adrenal tumour – surgical removal;

(3)   Cushing's disease:
   (a)   pituitary ablation or removal;
   (b)   adrenal blocking drugs such as metyrapone;

(4)   Congenital adrenal hyperplasia – suppression with dexamethasone or predisone in monitored dosage taken at night;

(5)   Severe hirsutism:
   (a)   suppression of the ovary with an oral contraceptive preparation cyclically (marvelon);
   (b)   suppression of the adrenal with dexamethasone or prednisone 5 mg, again taken at night, to block the early morning ACTH surge;
   (c)   antiandrogens such as cyproterone acetate taken cyclically with oestrogens and other measures to ensure that conception does not occur.

Following are the main points to note about regimens for hirsutism.

(1)   They are all only of limited effectiveness in some women.

(2)   Therapy must be continued for long periods if it is to work at all.

(3)   Bear in mind the effect on fertility of regimens that suppress the ovary.

(4)   Always bear in mind the need to ensure contraception when antiandrogens which will demasculinize a male fetus are used.

Symptomatic treatment is very important in hirsutism.

(1)   Electrolysis is advised for the face. It must be by a skilled person.

(2)   Bleaching is useful for facial and body hair to make it less noticeable.

(3)   Plucking – only for a few hairs in non-painful areas.

(4)   Depilatory substances are useful for the legs.

(5)   Shaving – useful – but resisted, particularly for the face, because of a belief that it makes hair grow more quickly and also because of connotations of male behaviour patterns.

(6)   Cosmetic camouflage.

Information to patient/family

(1)   It is very important to work to produce realistic expectations for the treatment of hirsutism. Many women even with significant hirsutism would be better advised to accept the problem rather than go through prolonged courses of relatively ineffective treatment involving attendance at endocrine clinics which can alter their perception of themselves as normal women. Helpful advice on symptomatic measures and reassurance are often effective. Very often the real problem is a fear that the sexual partner will be repelled but only rarely has the topic been openly discussed. This can be the most effective therapy of all when a woman realizes she is loved for herself and that the partner does not actually care about the hirsuitism.

(2)   Information about suppression of the ovary and possible effects on future fertility must be given before treatment.

(3) The risks of antiandrogens must be explained.

(4) It should be explained that the woman is not changing sex. This is a common and commonly expressed fear, particularly in teenagers.

Prevention

There are no effective prevention measures other than careful use of oral progestogens and other drugs with androgen actions.

After care

Considerable long term support may be required for women with serious hirsutism. Women on antiandrogens must be carefully monitored by the endocrinologist.

DISORDERS OF SEXUAL DIFFERENTIATION

What are they?

The term refers to abnormalities of sexual development usually detected by the appearance of the genitalia in newborn or very young children.

There are three main groups to consider:

(1) The female child who is virilized – usually owing to congenital adrenal hyperplasia (CAH).

(2) The male child who is incompletely virilized or developed – usually owing to androgen receptor deficits.

(3) Intersex appearance with some features of both sexes – often due to chromosome anomalies.

Problems

These are always extremely specialized problems and should always be referred immediately.

Clinical features

(1) In the virilized female with CAH there is an enlarged clitoris often with poor development of the labia and lower vagina.

(2) In the incompletely virilized male child there is usually a more normal male perineum with varying degrees of hypospadias or clefting of the scrotum.

(3) Intersex appearances by definition are confusing.

Assessment and investigation

These are very specialized. CAH can be detected as previously described.

Management

Clearly the decision as to which sex to rear such a child is crucial. Girls with CAH are reared appropriately. Some (chromosomally) male children with severely deficient masculinization or intersex also are better reared as girls. The decision is very specialized.

Information to family

It is of the utmost importance that this is approached uniformly after specialist advice. Clearly many problems can be expected in the future in relation to puberty and sexual relationships.

ENDOCRINE EFFECTS OF OVARIAN TUMOURS

What are they?

Most ovarian tumours are non-functioning endocrinologically. Those that do function are shown in Table 13. In addition tumours commonly arise in dysgenetic gonads and are either functioning or silent. At high risk are those with XO/XY or XO/XX mosaics and people with paragonadal dysgenesis.

Table 13 Endocrine effects of ovarian tumours

Endocrine effects	Tumour type	Usual presentation	Hormone secreted
Feminizing	Granulosa cell Theca cell Teratomata	A young woman with erratic menses and heavy bleeding Rarely precocious puberty	Oestrodiol Rarely progesterone Teratomata secreting HCG rarely
Masculinizing	Arrhenoblastoma Hilus cell adenoma Adrenal cell rests	A pelvic mass Amenorrhoea plus hirsutism and virilization	Testosterone Adrenal rests may also secrete cortisol and oestrogens
Thyroid	Struma ovarii (teratomatous)	Very very rare Cause of thyrotoxicosis	Thyroid hormones

Assessment and investigations

The main thing is to bear such tumours in mind in any female with:

(1)   precocious puberty,
(2)   heavy erratic menses,
(3)   hirsutism and menstrual irregularity.

A pelvic assessment is the first priority with appropriate further investigation if a mass is found. The appropriate endocrine investigations can be presumed from the information on Table 13.

Management

This is surgical.

ENDOCRINE DISORDERS OF THE BREAST

Failure to develop

This is discussed under hypogonadism and puberty . Congenital absence may occur (one or both) and the nipple may be absent.

Abnormalities

Asymmetry of breasts and accessory breasts and nipples occur more frequently and cause concern. Surgery may be needed.

PAINFUL BREASTS (CHRONIC MASTITIS)

What is it?

There is a chronic state of pain usually accompanied by swelling and eventually diffuse nodular change. The pain is usually worse premenstrually and the syndrome abates after the menopause. It may be exacerbated by oral contraceptives.

Problems

The condition causes a great deal of distress to women.

It is difficult to treat.

There is often (unspoken) fear of cancer.

Cancer may coexist.

Clinical features

The breasts are tender to palpation. They may feel normal or diffusely shotty and nodular. There may be a definite lump – tender or not tender – or multiple lumps.

Assessment

Every lump in the breast should be assessed independently on its merits because of the possibility of carcinoma. Aspiration needle or open biopsy may be needed and mammography can be helpful in differentiation.

Management

This is difficult. Any of the following may give relief:

(1)   A supporting brassiere (also at night)
(2)   Stopping oral oestrogens
(3)   A trial of oral contraceptives
(4)   Diuretics
(5)   Danazol 200 mg b.d.
(6)   Bromocriptine

Reassurance about cancer is often effective.

GALACTORRHOEA

What is it?

Galactorrhoea is the persistent discharge of milk from either female or male breast.

Causes

These are shown in Table 14.

Table 14   Causes of galactorrhoea

Pituitary tumour – a prolactinoma may be a microadenoma
Drugs
  – oestrogens, e.g. 'the pill'
  – phenothiazines
  – tricyclic antidepressants
Suckling reflex
  – previous herpes zoster
  – thoracic surgery
  – persistent breast feeding
  – excess manipulation of the breasts
Hypothyroidism
Bronchial carcinoma with ectopic prolactin secretion

There is usually but not always elevation of serum prolactin due to oversecretion, or lack or prolactin inhibitory factor.

Problems

(1)   Galactorrhoea may be milky (white) or serous (clear fluid).

(2)   Coloured or bloodstained discharges from the nipple usually indicate chronic mastitis or intraduct carcinoma and require appropriate investigation.

(3) The condition can cause distress.

(4) It may be associated with amenorrhoea and infertility or impotence in men.

Clinical features

A woman may complain of discharge or be unaware of it.

Always check for galactorrhoea by expressing the breast if a woman complains of amenorrhoea.

Assessment and investigations

(1) Exclude coloured or bloodstained discharges;

(2) Exclude pregnancy or recent pregnancy;

(3) Serial prolactin estimations to confirm elevation;

(4) Pituitary fossa tomography to define a tumour or micro-adenoma;

(5) Serum T4 and TSH estimations to exclude hypothyroidism;

(6) Drug screen now and usage in the past. A period of amenor-rhoea or oligomenorrhoea may date from use of an oral contraceptive for 6 months, 2 or 3 years earlier;

(7) Chest X-ray – a carcinoma will require treatment;

(8) If a pituitary tumour is present this will need assessment;

(9) If the prolactin level is normal, check for persistent breast manipulation.

Management

Specific

(1) Pituitary tumour may require treatment.

(2) Bromocriptine starting with 2.5 mg nocte or b.d. will suppress the prolactin level. Continue treatment for 6 months.

(3) Hypothyroidism should be treated.

Symptomatic

Advice to leave the breasts strictly alone should always be given. No looking to see if it is still there.

Information to patient

(1) Advise that treatment with bromocriptine will probably induce a sudden return of fertility must always be given so that unwanted pregnancy can be avoided.

(2) Give reassurance that this is a common condition and not dangerous.

(3) Explanation of the connection between amenorrhoea or impotence, X-rays of the head and the milky discharge should be given. Excess prolactin secretion causes a state of hypogonadism by suppression of gonadotrophic hormone production and by an inhibitory ovarian action. Excess prolactin can come from a tumour of the pituitary which is almost never malignant but needs careful assessment periodically and possibly an operation or other direct treatment. Excess prolactin can be produced by drugs which suppress its inhibitory control factor or by stimulation of the 'suckling reflex'.

Prevention

Attention should be given to:

(1) misuse of oral contraceptives.
(2) overuse of other 'major' psychotropic drugs, and
(3) early diagnosis of hypothyroidism.

After care

If a pituitary tumour is present it will require long term assessment and follow-up with coordination of care from several specialists.

Bromocriptine should be given for a sufficient period (usually 6 months) to prevent relapses, which should always be checked for.

GYNAECOMASTIA

What is it?

Gynaecomastia is enlargement of the male breast.

Causes of gynaecomastia

These are summarized in Table 15.

What problems?

(1) In young people considerable distress can be caused and social difficulties particularly in connection with swimming occur.

(2) It may be difficult on occasions to distinguish 'true' enlargement of the duct and lobular tissue of the breast from 'false' gynaecomastia due to adipose deposits – particularly in older people.

(3) Despite all the 'causes' it is frequent not to find a cause or any hormonal change.

Clinical features

(1) The degree of enlargement varies from a small cone of tissue to a complete breast. It may be unilateral or difficult to

Table 15 Causes of gynaecomastia

The newborn – intrauterine environment
Pubertal – 50% of boys but goes in a year usually
Testicular – Klinefelter's, orchitis, atrophy, tumours
Hypogonadism – from any cause
Other endocrine diseases – adrenal tumour, acromegaly, Graves's disease
Chronic liver disease – 'oestrogens'
Carcinoma of bronchus – ectopic hormone secretion
Drugs – oestrogens, androgens, spironolactone, digoxin, reserpine, chlorpromazine
Starvation
Von Recklinghausen's disease
Carcinoma of the breast

Pubertal gynaecomastia, which may be severe, is common. In young men look for evidence of testicular disease. In middle-aged men liver disease is common and bronchial carcinoma and testicular tumour should be excluded. In elderly men gynaecomastia induced by oestrogens for prostatic carcinoma and digoxin and spironolactone is seen frequently. Other causes are rare

distinguish from adiposity. There may rarely be a carcinoma or galactorrhoea.

(2) Take a careful drug history.

(3) Check for past testicular disease (orchitis, bilateral torsion) and past illnesses such as jaundice.

(4) Examine the testes carefully.

(5) Look for signs of liver disease, heart failure or bronchial carcinoma.

Investigations

On the whole, investigations are not helpful, as in most cases hormone levels are normal. The following are found, however:

(1) raised FSH and LH in Klinefelter's and testicular failure,
(2) low testosterone in hypogonadism,
(3) raised prolactin in pituitary tumour or chlorpromazine usage,
(3) raised oestrodiol in testicular or adrenal oestrogen secreting tumour or (not always) in chronic liver disease.

Occasionally skull X-ray (for pituitary fossa), liver or thyroid function tests can be helpful.

Management

Specific

(1) Surgery is indicated if the condition is severe or causing severe distress.

(2) Danazol (an antigonadotrophic) helps in some people.

(3) Treatment should be directed, where appropriate, at specific causes such as drugs.

133

Symptomatic

In pubertal cases simple reassurance is all that is required, together with advice to wear loose clothing.

Always reassure boys (and men) that they are not changing sex – this is a frequent fantasy.

6

THE TESTIS

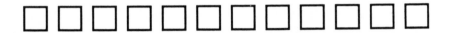

WHAT IS IT?

The testis is the male gonad. The mature testis in the adult is responsible for the production of spermatazoa and the secretion of testosterone. Sperm production occurs in the seminiferous tubules and it takes approximately 70 days for one mature sperm to form from the spermatogonium. Sperm in the testis achieves its fertility when passing through the epididymis attached to the testis. Further nutritional factors are added via secretion from the prostate during ejaculation.

Testosterone is produced from the Leydig cells in bursts of activity during the life span of a normal male. Dihydrotestosterone is a more potent natural androgen.

(1) Secretion of testosterone and dihydrotestosterone within the male fetus results in differentiation and development of the normal male genital tract. Failure of this mechanism may lead to various disorders of sexual differentiation. Tissue insensitivity to androgens results in the testicular feminization syndrome, a 'receptor disease' where the genotype is XY but the phenotype is female with normal breasts and external genitalia development and a blind vagina. Laparotomy of these individuals reveal testes in the abdomen or the inguinal canal.

(2)   Pubertal secretion. This is responsible for the development of secondary sexual characteristics and masculinization. Testosterone is carried in the blood to its target organs throughout the body. Ninety-five per cent of it is bound to sex hormone binding globulin and inactive. Its role throughout the body together with dihydrotestosterone is to maintain masculinization and also to contribute to the production of mature spermatozoa via its effect firstly on spermatogenesis and secondarily on prostate and seminal vesicle stimulation. Testosterone is metabolized in the liver and these metabolites appear in the form of 17-oxo steroids in the urine.

Testicular function is under the higher control of the pituitary and the hypothalamus. The pituitary produces follicle-stimulating hormone (FSH), the action of which contributes to the formation of sperm, and luteinizing hormone which stimulates testosterone production. High circulating levels of testosterone will inhibit release of luteinizing hormone by negative feedback and high circulating levels of inhibin from the seminiferous tubules will inhibit FSH release. Both these effects occur via the hypothalamus.

WHAT PROBLEMS?

(1)   Disorders of the testis are poorly understood, are often missed, are not easily treatable and are relatively uncommon in general practice.

(2)   Anxiety may be expressed about delay in secondary sexual changes at puberty which may be normal or indicate hypogonadism.

(3)   Infertility due to testicular causes accounts for approximately half the joint causation of infertility as a clinical problem for a couple.

(4)   Infertility in the male is not easily treated.

(5)   The hypogonad male is easily treated.

(6)   The conditions to be discussed in this chapter are hypogonadism, infertility and mechanical disorders.

HYPOGONADISM

Hypogonadism results in both infertility (*see below*) and lack of development or regression of secondary sexual characteristics, depending on whether the disorder commences before, during or after puberty.

Clinical features of hypogonadism are:

(1)   loss of sexual libido,

(2)   impotence,

(3)   small immature penis and testicles,

(4)   failure of development of or regression from male hair distribution patterns on face and body,

(5)   high pitched voice (only in hypogonadism coming on before puberty),

(6)   poor muscle development and gynaecomastia,

(7)   gynaecoid fat distribution,

(8)   abnormal skeletal proportions where the arm span is greater than the height and the pubis-to-floor height is greater than the pubis-to-crown height (this is called eunuchoid stature and only occurs in hypogonadism present during pubertal years).

Postpubertal changes of hypogonadism are more subtle and may present purely as loss of libido, infertility and mild regression of secondary sexual characteristics.

Causes of hypogonadism

The causes are either testicular or pituitohypothalamic.

The following list gives the commoner causes of primary testicular failure.

(1) Bilateral orchitis secondary to mumps or Coxsackie virus
(2) Post surgical trauma or other forms of castration
(3) Bilateral torsion
     Post radiation damage
     Varicocoele (more usually infertility alone)
     Chromosomal abnormalities, e.g. Klinefelter's syndrome
     Testicular agenesis

Secondary testicular failure usually occurs in conjunction with hypothalamopituitary disease and is due to gonadotrophin deficiency. It occurs:

(1) As part of generalized hypopituitarism,
(2) As isolated hypogonadotrophic hypogonadism (Kallman's syndrome),
(3) In 'delayed puberty' and
(4) In hyperprolactinaemic syndromes.

Investigation of the hypogonad man

As mentioned before, the most likely presentation is impotence or infertility and a careful history and examination is required to decide whether the cause is of primary testicular origin or secondary to hypothalamopituitary disease.

Helpful investigations in hypogonadism are as follows:

(1) Serum testosterone level is low in all causes.

(2) Serum FSH and LH:
    (a) high in testicular failure
    (b) low in hypothalamopituitary dysfunction.

(3) Serum prolactin is high in hyperprolactinaemic syndromes such as pituitary prolactinoma and associated with low gonadotrophins and sometimes gynaecomastia and galactorrhoea.

(4)   Sex chromosome studies.

(5)   Radiological bone age on wrist X-ray provides an index of skeletal maturity.

Management of hypogonadism

The first decision is whether to treat at all. Many hypogonad males do not wish to have their condition either investigated too far or localized. It is important to exclude space occupying pituitary lesions but otherwise management very much depends on the problems and wishes of the person and or the couple involved.

The important principles in endocrine management are as follows.

(1)   Primary testicular failure is treated with androgen replacement by testosterone analogues – by depot injection usually (e.g. Sustanon), but also by tablet or sublingually. Such treatment restores both libido and potency.

(2)   Hypothalamopituitary disease, once suspected, should be referred for expert assessment. Hypogonadism due to pituitary causes can be treated by androgen replacement but this will not induce spermatogenesis and, if a couple wishes, fertility treatment with gonadotrophins can be given by experts.

(3)   Hyperprolactinaemic syndromes can be readily treated with bromocriptine.

(4)   The impotent male: a detailed sexual history including the frequency of masturbation and nocturnal and early morning erections is important. Morning erections and masturbation often remain despite functional impotency. Current or previous illness and venereal disease should be asked about, as should the state of the main relationship and any other sexual outlets or sources of either resentment or guilt. Previous and present drug history is important, as is drug abuse – of tobacco, alcohol or other drugs.

(5) Delayed puberty: this is dealt with more fully in Chapter 5. The following should be noted:

    (a) The average time of onset of puberty for white males in the United Kingdom is 12 ± 2 years. Individuals who have not *started* puberty by 14 years of age are regarded as having delayed puberty and should be investigated.

    (b) Parental anxiety over delayed puberty is much commoner with boys. A family history is important in indicating expected time of onset of puberty. Enquire of the parents when their own puberty commenced. Intercurrent disease should be excluded – this is a common cause for delayed onset of adolescence.

Case history

A 48-year-old man presented with a troublesome seborrhoeic dermatitis of the scalp and was seen over a period of months. He was noted also to have rather fine facial hair growth, soft voice and female hairline. Absence of hair on arms and hands were also observed. On subsequent assessment of his scalp condition he was questioned about his past history. He denied ever having any problems with sexual intercourse although he had been divorced for some 10 years and there was no issue from his marriage. He said his hair growth had always been light. He was willing to be further examined and when undressed revealed some degree of gynaecomastia and a somewhat female pelvic fat distribution. He had absent axillary hair and a female pubic escutcheon. The penis was small as were his testes and scrotum. Crude assessment of his visual fields was normal and there were no obvious stigmata or other endocrine anomalies.

I thought the most likely diagnosis here was Klinefelter's syndrome but as he was complaining of his dandruff and not of his general appearance I declined to investigate him further. What other tests might I have done without upsetting him too much which might have helped to confirm or deny my diagnosis?

THE INFERTILE MALE

Clinical features

The clinical features of infertility either are those of hypogonadism or are limited to the finding of anatomical abnormalities of the testes, or are absent. The testes and scrotum should always be carefully examined in the infertile man. There may be:

(1) absent testes,
(2) cryptorchidism,
(3) small testes,
(4) varicocoele.

Cryptorchidism

This deserves a brief mention here since it is important to evaluate the undescended testis early in life, and distinguish it from the retractile testis which is harmless. Any testicle which cannot be palpated in the scrotum or coaxed into the scrotum by genital manipulation must be referred to a specialist, since undescended testicles lead to subsequent subfertility even when detected at the age of 5 years and there is an increased incidence of malignant change in the undescended testicle.

Small testes

Since 99% of the bulk of the testis is made up of seminiferous tubules, any testicular insult such as mumps or orchitis tends to reduce the testicular size. The understimulated testis of pituitary disease is soft and lacks characteristic pain sensation on pressure. The testis in Klinefelter's syndrome is characteristically *very* small (minute up to the size of a pea).

Varicocoele

Varicocoele is common and may contribute to or cause infertility.

141

The following are worthy of note:

(1) Surgical correction of varicocoele may improve sperm counts but should only be attempted when the varicocoele is large and symptomatic;

(2) Results of varicocoele surgery on subsequent conception rates are not so impressive as results on sperm counts.

Investigation of the infertile man

Infertility is the problem of a couple and should always be investigated as such, with properly organized tests on both partners with results readily accessible to all (*see also* Chapter 5). Many problems, such as primarily sexual problems or rocky relationships, inappropriate designation of blame etc, are also missed if couples are not seen together. In addition many men try to avoid infertility investigations, preferring to believe that barrenness is a failing of women. This is not the case. It is emotionally extremely wearing to go through infertility investigations and the subsequent seesaw of monthly expectations. Even though it is unusual to be able to do much for the sperm count of men with fertility problems, in some you can – but in all, the support and involvement of the man is of paramount importance.

The sperm count

This is extremely variable between individuals and different laboratories. A rough guide is as follows:

Volume: between 1 and 6 ml.
Motility should be greater than 60% after 3 hours.
Sperm count should be greater than 20×10^6 ml.
Morphology shows greater than 60% sperms normal.
Fructose should also be present if tested for. It is an indication of prostatic secretion.

A fresh specimen should be produced by masturbation and analysed. If the count is in doubt, at least three specimens should be taken with several days interlude between, to allow time to gain maximum density.

The causes of low sperm count or azoospermia are:

(1) any cause of hypogonadism,
(2) absent or undescended testes,
(3) venereal disease,
(4) cytotoxic drugs,
(5) irradiation to the testis,
(6) varicocoele.

Testicular biopsy is sometimes of benefit either in demonstrating absent germinal epithelium, the degree of spermatogenic arrest or the fact that the testis is normal and swollen with sperm. This can indicate blockage of the ductal apparatus.

Always investigate for associated hypogonadism and hyperprolactinaemia.

MANAGEMENT

About 5 % of men with infertility can be specifically treated. These include:

(1) hyperprolactinaemia (with bromocriptine),
(2) hypopituitarism (with gonadotrophin therapy),
(3) rare ductal blockage syndromes,
(4) a few with low sperm counts by various therapeutic regimes.

However most spermatozoa are killed by vaginal secretions before reaching the endocervix and measures including artificial insemination by husband (AIH) are available which can increase the effective sperm count enormously.

THE IMPOTENT MALE

Sexual impotence implies the inability to achieve sexual intercourse by sustained erection and ejaculation. The differentiation between organic and functional impotence is important.

Vasectomy

Vasectomy deserves a brief mention here as it is an increasingly common request and a good explanation of what the surgery involves, and what the after-effects may be, is required. This should be the role of every family doctor. There are handouts specifically for this given by the UK Health Education Council. It can be quite an uncomfortable operation and there may be problems with intercourse afterwards, so that counselling may be required. Always stress that it takes at least 3 months for the male to become sterile after vasectomy and that follow-up sperm counts should be sent to the laboratory until sterility has been proved. Individuals are notoriously bad at producing specimens after the event. Vasectomy can be surgically reversed but conception rates are low, possibly because in the meantime sperm antibodies have been produced which effectively render the sperm infertile.

ANATOMICAL DISORDERS OF THE TESTIS

These can be considered under three headings.

(1)   Maldescent of the testis
(2)   Testicular pain
(3)   Testicular lump

Maldescent

The testis develops from the genital fold on the posterior abdominal wall and descends to the scrotum normally by birth under the influence of the gubernaculum. Problems can be:

(1)   Incomplete descent – the testis does not lie in the scrotum but is on the correct path, and

144

(2) Ectopic testis – the testis has followed an inappropriate route of descent.

Management should not be delayed. First distinguish incomplete descent from retractile testis (as mentioned above). Orchidopexy should be offered certainly before the age of 5. It is very likely that maldescent occurs when there is some pre-existing, possibly genetic, anomaly of the testis. There is a very high infertility rate in maldescent even when the testis is brought down early and even when it is unilateral.

Testicular pain

Severe testicular pain occurs in torsion, acute epididymo-orchitis (often due to coliform infection), acute orchitis (often due to mumps) and trauma. If there is any doubt, surgical exploration is indicated as a matter of urgency to exclude torsion.

The testicular lump

This is the most likely presentation of testicular problems in family practice. It is important to try and distinguish between hydrocoele, epididymal cyst, varicocoele, hernia, orchitis, torsion, tumour and granuloma. Only the varicocoele is a potentially reversible cause of male infertility. Tumours are usually painless. They are almost all malignant. They are hard and there may be associated lymphadenopathy. Some testicular tumours (teratomas) produce hormones such as HCG which may cause gynaecomastia. Early referral to a specialist is indicated. The results of chemotherapy and radiation on teratoma and seminoma are now exceedingly good and the morbidity has been considerably reduced over the past 15 years.

7

DISEASES OF THE PITUITARY

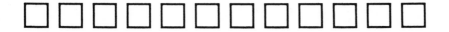

WHAT ARE THEY?

Disorders of the pituitary gland can be considered under three main headings:

(1) Hypopituitarism

(2) Syndromes resulting from excess secretion of pituitary gland hormones

(3) Space occupying lesions in the pituitary fossa

Firstly, some information about the pituitary gland and its functions.

THE PITUITARY GLAND

The anterior and posterior pituitary glands lie within the bony sella turcica or pituitary fossa at the base of the brain. The anterior pituitary is formed from Rathke's pouch, an invagination of the oral region. The posterior pituitary is an outpouching of neural tissue from the floor of the III ventricle. The hypothalamus lies around the III ventricle above the pituitary and next to the optic chiasm. It consists of well-defined nuclei and tracts,

147

(1)   supraoptic nuclei,
(2)   paraventricular nuclei,

the cells of which secrete the posterior pituitary hormones:

(1)   Vasopressin (the antidiuretic hormone),
(2)   Oxytocin (stimulates uterine contractions; function unclear), and their specific binding proteins known as neurophysins. These pass down the axons of the neurons down the hypothalamic-neurohypophyseal tract, being finally secreted into capillaries in the posterior pituitary.

Nuclei in the basal hypothalamus also secrete specific releasing and inhibiting hormones, as follows:

(1)   Thyrotrophin releasing hormone (TRH), also releases prolactin.

(2)   Gonadotrophin releasing hormone (LHRH) releases both LH and FSH.

(3)   Corticotrophin releasing factor (CRF) releases ACTH – structure not known.

(4)   Growth hormone release inhibiting hormone (somatostatin) – lowers GH levels. Also reduces insulin, glucagon and gastrin levels.

(5)   Prolactin inhibiting factor (may be dopamine) inhibits prolactin.

(6)   Other less well-defined factors (e.g. growth hormone releasing hormone).

The ability of TRH and LHRH when injected intravenously to raise serum levels of the appropriate hormones is used clinically in TRH and LHRH tests of the hypothalamo-pituitary axis. Hypothalamic releasing hormones/pituitary trophic hormones/ target endocrine gland hormones form a cascade amplifying system by means of which minute quantities of releasing hormones allow control of much larger quantities of target hormones. There is a very delicate feedback system operating at hypothalamic and pituitary levels. As stated, releasing and inhibiting hormones control the activity of the anterior pituitary. Efferent nerve fibres from the basal hypothalamus join the hypothalamo-hypophyseal tract ending in the portal veins. The releasing hormones are secreted by these neurons and travel to the anterior pituitary via the portal veins.

The hormones secreted by the anterior pituitary are:

(1) growth hormone (GH),
(2) thyroid stimulating hormone (TSH),
(3) adrenocorticotrophic hormone (ACTH),
(4) luteinizing hormone (LH),
(5) follicle stimulating hormone (FSH),
(6) prolactin.

Their actions and regulation are summarized in Table 16.

HYPOPITUITARISM

What is it?

Several syndromes can be recognized, as follows.

(1) Panhypopituitarism (Simmonds's disease) – usually a chronic illness with variable deficiency of most of the anterior pituitary hormones. A severe form exists. Usually caused by pituitary tumour. Also occurs after surgery or DXT, as postpartum necrosis (Sheehan's syndrome) or due to granulomatous lesions. Sheehan's syndrome is now very rare.

(2) Diabetes insipidus – due to absence of vasopressin and is sometimes seen with panhypopituitarism, particularly after surgery, but also occurs alone commonly after head trauma or surgery and in granulomatous conditions (sarcoid, histiocytosis etc).

(3) Isolated deficiencies of particular pituitary hormones as occur for instance in isolated hypogonadotrophic

149

Table 16 Anterior pituitary hormones

Hormone	Actions	Regulation
Growth hormone. A polypeptide	Growth in children. Metabolic actions throughout life (mobilizes FFA; increases amino acid uptake into protein) GH stimulation of protein synthesis cartilage is mediated by somatomedin from the liver	Pulsatile release particularly during sleep. Exercise and stress and hypoglycaemia raise levels. Hyperglycaemia suppresses
Thyroid stimulating hormone. A glycoprotein	Thyroid stimulation synthesis and release of thyroid hormones	Negative feedback from thyroid hormones
Adrenocorticotrophic hormone. A polypeptide derived from the same cells as β-endorphin and pro-γ-MSH	Stimulates adrenal cortex to produce cortisol and adrenal androgens	Negative feedback from cortisol. Also a diurnal rhythm. Also stress and hypoglycaemia stimulate cortisol production

Luteinizing hormone. A glycoprotein Follicle stimulating hormone. A glycoprotein	Both act in the female to promote ovarian growth and oestrogen secretion. FSH is more important in follicular development. LH surge causes ovulation. In the male FSH is largely concerned with spermatogenesis, LH with stimulation of androgen production from Leydig cells	Gonadotroph secretion varies. It is low in infancy, rises through puberty, shows complex patterns in the adult state and rises in later life. In adults there is pulsatile release particularly of LH and in the female episodic gonadotroph release in the menstrual cycle particularly a midcycle peak of LH which triggers ovulation. In postmenopausal women FSH and LH levels are high, as they are to some extent in older men. Testosterone suppresses LH production. Oestrogens suppress FSH in the female but have first negative and then positive effects on LH. FSH levels are lowered by inhibin from the graafian follicle and seminiferous tubule
Prolactin. A polypeptide	In the female stimulates breast growth and milk production. Role in man is unknown. High prolactin levels interfere with gonadotroph production and their gonadal actions	Prolactin is a 'stress' hormone – levels rise in emotion and on exercise. Prolactin is under tonic inhibiting control. Breast stimulation increases prolactin levels

hypogonadism (Kallman's syndrome), where it is associated with anosmia, but also noted with TSH, GH and ACTH.

In pituitary tumour GH and LH and FSH are often lost before TSH and ACTH.

What problems?

(1) Hypopituitarism is often of insidious onset and chronic course. The symptoms are similar to depression and the condition is often missed.

(2) Assessment of pituitary disease requires multiple specialists, very often inpatient care and prolonged follow-up. Coordination of care is often a major problem.

(3) Treatment again requires prolonged monitoring.

(4) Hypopituitarism should never be assessed without simultaneous assessment of the pituitary fossa for tumour etc.

Clinical features

These depend on the particular hormone deficits and the time of life.

(1) GH: In children, failure to grow. In adults, very little effect.

(2) TSH: A partial degree of hypothyroidism often greater in children.

(3) ACTH: Symptoms of hypoadrenalism, in particular lethargy, anorexia, weakness. A finding of hypoglycaemia. Little electrolyte disturbance (compare Addison's disease) due to intact renin–aldosterone system. Absence of pigmentation (cf. Addison's disease).

(4) Gonadotrophs: In childhood or adolescence there will be failure of pubertal development, partial or total. In adults

there will be amenorrhoea, breast atrophy, loss of pubic and axillary hair, loss of potency and libido and infertility.

(5)   Prolactin: Failure of lactation in adults.

Clinical clues to hypopituitarism are:

(1)   Pale wrinkled skin

(2)   Lack of axillary hair

(3)   Amenorrhoea or impotence (enquire)

Assessment and investigations

The hormonal assessment given is not enough – the pituitary fossa and visual systems must be checked also (*see* pituitary tumour, p. 166). Endocrine investigations are done to determine the extent of hormone deficits. This can usually be done in a single morning using a combined test of pituitary function. This does not require admission to hospital but is best done in a hospital day ward or metabolic ward. Insulin hypoglycaemia tests should never be done by those inexperienced in their use.

Combined test of anterior pituitary function

This is shown in Table 17.

Management

Specific

Hormone replacement may be given as follows.

(1)   Cortisol (20–30 mg/day) or prednisone (5–8 mg day) for adrenal replacement. Increase in times of stress. Mineralocorticoids are not required.

153

(2) Thyroxine – monitor dosage on serum levels.

(3) GH – given by injection to children. Not needed for adults.

(4) If fertility is not an issue, give testosterone esters by intramuscular injection monthly to males and an oral contraceptive preparation to women. Fertility can be induced with FSH and HCG injections and sometimes with LHRH.

Table 17   Combined test of anterior pituitary function

Basal	Stimulation tests (done simultaneously)
Cortisol GH	Insulin induced hypoglycaemia: Serial 15 minute samples for 2 hours for cortisol and GH
TSH T4 Prolactin	TRH tests: 20 and 60 minute samples for TSH and prolactin after i.v. injection of TRH
LH FSH Testosterone or oestrodiol	LHRH tests: 20 and 60 minute samples for LH and FSH after i.v. injection of LHRH
Sometimes ACTH	

Information to patient/family

There are several points to be made.

(1) Necessity for continued attention and prolonged follow-up particularly for those on partial replacement only.

(2) Steroid instructions. A steroid card should always be made out and instruction given to double the steroid dose temporarily when illness strikes. If vomiting occurs parenteral administration of steroids may be needed.

(3) It should be stressed that normal health is the rule on replacement therapy.

Prevention

Better obstetric care has reduced the incidence of Sheehan's syndrome. Increased awareness on the part of the doctor of the presentation and clinical features of hypopituitarism may prevent progression and late diagnosis.

After care

As stated, repeated clinical assessment and estimation of hormone levels are necessary, together with repeated assessments of vision and the pituitary fossa if a tumour is involved. There is a role for the GP – co-ordinating and maintaining these various follow-up necessities.

DIABETES INSIPIDUS

This usually only occurs with damage to the upper pituitary stalk or hypothalamus, as previously detailed. Many cases are without definable cause, and remember there is a nephrogenic variety.

What problems?

(1) It is often difficult to be sure of the extent of 'polyuria' without hospitalization.

(2) Psychogenic polydipsia is commoner than true diabetes insipidus.

Clinical features

(1) Polyuria due to inability to concentrate the urine leads to thirst with compensatory polydipsia.

(2) Severe cases very easily become severely dehydrated.

155

(3) The condition is often transient after head surgery or injury.

Assessment and investigations

It is important to consider other causes of polyuria:

(1) psychogenic polydipsia,
(2) diabetes mellitus,
(3) chronic renal failure,
(4) hypercalcaemia,
(5) hypokalaemia,
(6) diuretic abuse and
(7) lithium therapy.

Usually the differentiation of diabetes insipidus from psychogenic polydipsia requires hospitalization to

(1) document the degree of polyuria,
(2) perform a water deprivation test,
(3) establish responsiveness to vasopressin and determine the correct dose.

Water deprivation test

This is a complicated procedure with many pitfalls for the inexperienced. It involves serial measurements of plasma and urine osmolality, body weight and urine volume in which the patient is denied fluids for a period – either until body weight drops by 5% (say 3 kg) or a 12-hour maximum period. Those with diabetes insipidus start with a high plasma osmolality and lose weight with continued urine production. Psychogenic polydipsia gives a low basal plasma osmolality and on dehydration urine volumes fall.

Management

Vasopressin tannate in oil has now been superseded by either

156

synthetic lysine vasopressin or the long acting desmopressin (DDAVP) which is given nasally once or twice a day.

After care

Prolonged follow-up is necessary, with checks of serum sodium concentration to guard against overtreatment (low levels).

SYNDROMES RESULTING FROM EXCESS SECRETION OF PITUITARY HORMONES

These syndromes are as follows.

(1) Acromegaly resulting from excess secretion of GH from an eosinophil adenoma of the pituitary. This in young people will produce gigantism.

(2) Cushing's disease: a disturbance of the feedback control of cortisol production resulting in excess ACTH levels and high cortisol levels. This results in bilateral adrenal hyperplasia and basophil adenoma (often microadenomata) of the pituitary.

(3) Hyperprolactinaemia: seen physiologically in pregnancy and lactation. The most common pathological cause is a pituitary adenoma (often microadenomata). It can also occur in hypothyroidism, acromegaly and after surgery or trauma to the pituitary. Drugs, particularly oestrogens and phenothiazines, can cause high prolactin levels.

ACROMEGALY

What problems?

(1) This is a disease of insidious onset and slow course, often late diagnosed.

(2) Treatments available are generally invasive which has led in the past to delay in treating known cases.

(3) Acromegaly does however shorten life, causing death by cardiovascular and diabetic conditions (diabetes occurs as a complication in about 25%) and should be effectively treated.

Clinical features

Excess growth hormone in the adult can no longer cause increased height, as the epiphyses have fused, but the following do result:

(1) Skeletal enlargement of the head, jaw (prognathism), hands and feet,

(2) Soft tissue enlargement giving spade-like hands, thick coarse skin, enlargement of the lips and tongue, nerve entrapment (carpal tunnel syndrome),

(3) Visceromegaly – enlargement of the kidneys, heart etc,

(4) A specific acromegalic cardiomyopathy and hypertension and

(5) Diabetes in 25%, as GH is an insulin antagonist.

In addition, features of a pituitary tumour are present (*see below*); the tumour is often characteristically large. One of these features often seen in acromegaly is the development of hypopituitarism due presumably to pressure by the tumour on normally functioning pituitary tissue.

Assessment and investigations

The essential thing is to think of it. The crucial test for acromegaly is the finding of elevated growth hormone (GH) levels that do not suppress during a glucose tolerance test. Random GH values are hardly worth obtaining since levels are elevated by stress and exercise. The following are useful:

(1) X-ray evidence of a large pituitary fossa,
(2) Widening of the joint spaces due to cartilaginous overgrowth,
(3) Increased heel pad thickness on X-ray, and
(4) Biochemically a high serum phosphate level is seen in active acromegaly.

Specific management

Acromegaly shortens life and active intervention is indicated.

(1) Bromocriptine therapy lowers GH levels in acromegaly (it elevates them in normal people). A partial response is normally seen and the long term benefit is probably not as great as was hoped when this drug was originally introduced.

(2) An attack on the pituitary gland is usually more definitive and this can take the following forms.

    (a) *Surgery* – Transfrontal hypophysectomy is usually indicated when there is a suprasellar extension of the tumour with or without compression of the optic chiasm.

       Trans-sphenoidal hypophysectomy is undertaken increasingly for the removal of smaller tumours, of microadenomata and sometimes for tumours with small suprasellar extensions according to the experience of the operator.

    (b) *Radiotherapy* – Some centres are skilled in the implantation of radioactive yttrium or gold seeds. Heavy particle therapy also can be quite successful but is available at only very few centres. External X-ray therapy is usually not particularly successful.

The index of successful response to therapy is lowered growth hormone levels. Clinical response can be dramatic with regression of soft tissue changes, amelioration in hypertension and diabetes and lowered mortality.

159

Information to patient and family

(1) Always by discreet questioning exclude the possibility of multiple endocrine adenomatosis – in which condition endocrine disease is often seen in more than one member of the family or in more than one gland system. Pituitary, parathyroid and gastrin-secreting tumours are common.

(2) Acromegaly alters appearance and so can affect relationships and feelings. Careful handling of both the person affected and his near relatives is important.

(3) It is necessary to point out that effective therapy is usually surgical and causes some risk but that the likelihood of a good response is high.

(4) The question of subsequent fertility should be considered in those people undergoing pituitary gland surgery.

After care

Prolonged follow-up is necessary in acromegaly to:

(1) assess clinical and biochemical response to treatment,
(2) monitor the development of hypopituitarism, and
(3) monitor the replacement therapy.

CUSHING'S DISEASE

Cushing's syndrome is attributable to excess secretion of adrenal hormones particularly cortisol and occurs as follows:

(1) Cushing's disease – due to a disturbance of hypothalamic feedback control of cortisol. This results in overproduction of ACTH from the pituitary.

(2) Adenoma or carcinoma of the adrenal.

(3) Ectopic production of ACTH by tumours (e.g. bronchial carcinoma).

(4)   Administration of steroid medicines.

Here only the first will be dealt with. Clinical features of all 4 kinds are similar though there are differences (*see* Chapter 8, on the adrenal glands).

What problems?

(1)   Cushing's is of insidious onset and is often missed early in its course.

(2)   Many people with simple obesity are referred to hospital for investigation of Cushing's.

(3)   The full investigation of Cushing's is complex and involves admission to hospital, and should only be undertaken in those who clinically are thought to have a reasonable chance of having the condition.

(4)   Treatment for Cushing's disease is unsatisfactory.

Clinical features

These are discussed in Chapter 8.

Assessment and investigations

(1)   Firstly look for the clinical features of Cushing's syndrome – in particular thin arms and legs, easy bruising and proximal myopathy.

(2)   A short dexamethasone suppression test is a useful screening investigation when Cushing's is suspected clinically. This is described in Chapter 8 and can easily be performed in general practice.

(3)   When Cushing's syndrome is suspected as a result of points (1) and (2), then inpatient investigation is required.

There are two main aims:

(1) confirm excess cortisol production,
(2) determine the source.

Cortisol production

Plasma and urinary cortisol measurements and plasma ACTH measurements have replaced older measurements of urinary steroid metabolites. The following are found:

(1) There are elevated morning and evening plasma cortisol levels with loss of diurnal rhythm.

(2) In Cushing's disease the plasma cortisol is suppressible with 8 mg a day (2 mg 6-hourly) of dexamethasone but not by 2 mg a day (0.5 mg 6-hourly).

(3) In all other causes the plasma cortisol is not suppressible even by 8 mg of dexamethasone per day.

(4) The plasma ACTH is high in Cushing's disease, very high in ectopic ACTH production and suppressed in adrenal tumour and exogenous steroid administration.

(5) 24 h urinary cortisol secretion is a useful measurement.

Localizing the source

The following investigations can be helpful:

(1) X-ray of pituitary fossa – usually normal even in Cushing's disease but can show a microadenoma or occasionally even a definite 'basophil adenoma';

(2) CAT scan of the head – can be normal;

(3) Adrenal imaging techniques including:
     (a) intravenous urography (i.v.u.)
     (b) adrenal angiography

162

(c)   adrenal isotope scans (radiolabelled cholesterol)

(d)   CAT scan of adrenal area

(4)   X-ray evidence of ectopic ACTH producing tumour, e.g. chest X-ray.

Specific management

There is no widely accepted single therapy for Cushing's disease. Treatment must be undertaken, however, as the prognosis untreated is poor.

(1)   The condition is best treated by an attack on the pituitary.

Microadenomata of the basophil type are commonly found though large tumours are rare. Hypophysectomy is probably the treatment of choice, usually trans-sphenoidally.

(2)   Bilateral adrenalectomy can be undertaken. It is a major surgical procedure. It should be followed by radiotherapy to the pituitary to prevent Nelson's syndrome – a condition of rapidly growing pituitary tumour commonly with visual damage which occurs after adrenalectomy for Cushing's disease in 10% of people.

(3)   If available, yttrium implanation or heavy particle radiation may be successful, or even conventional radiation can be tried.

(4)   Medical treatment with adrenal blocking drugs such as aminoglutethimide, metyrapone or trilostane can be tried either to 'prepare' people for surgery or for people with untreatable adrenal tumours etc to ameliorate the metabolic effects.

Information to patient and/or family

It is important that the disease is put into context for the sufferer

163

and his or her family. The investigations for Cushing's syndrome are time consuming and often not definitive. Multiple admissions to hospital are often necessary before therapy – which can be of an invasive nature – is undertaken. It is important that the risks and reasons are understood.

After care

Prolonged after care is necessary because of:

(1)   the possibility of a pituitary tumour particularly after bilateral adrenalectomy,

(2)   the monitoring of effects of therapy,

(3)   the monitoring of steroid replacement therapy.

HYPERPROLACTINAEMIA

What problems?

(1)   Not all those with hyperprolactinaemia will have clinical evidence of this state. It is therefore necessary to screen for prolactin elevation in all men presenting with infertility and impotence, and all women with amenorrhoea.

(2)   Prolactin elevation is frequently intermittent. A single elevated level does not confirm pathology and a single normal value does not exclude it.

Clinical features

(1)   Due to the action of prolactin previously mentioned these are:

    (a)   impotence and infertility in men – occasionally galactorrhoea,

    (b)   amenorrhoea and infertility in women – galactorrhoea in about a third.

(2) There may be features of a pituitary tumour.

(3) There may be features of hypothyroidism acromegaly or a history of taking oestrogens or phenothiazines.

Assessment and investigations

(1) At least three determinations of serum prolactin (normal <270 iu/l (men) and <600 iu/l (women)).

(2) Investigation appropriate to a pituitary tumour including CAT scan of the pituitary.

(3) Screen for drugs appropriately.

(4) Exclude hypothyroidism.

Specific management

(1) A pituitary tumour or microadenoma is best treated by surgery with or without pituitary irradiation.

(2) Bromocriptine is very helpful for those with normal pituitary fossae.

(3) Treat any hypothyroidism or acromegaly.

Information to patient and family

It is essential before giving bromocriptine to inform the patient that contraception is necessary if desired, since fertility may be restored within days.

Prevention

Avoid misuse of oestrogens and major tranquillizers.

After care

After care is that appropriate to any pituitary tumour.

SPACE OCCUPYING LESION IN THE PITUITARY FOSSA

The endocrinological effects of a pituitary tumour must always be considered separately from any effects due to a space occupying lesion in the fossa. The causes of space occupying lesions in the region of the pituitary are shown in Table 18.

Table 18   Some causes of a space occupying lesion in the pituitary fossa

Chromophobe adenoma
Prolactinoma
Growth hormone secreting (eosinophil) adenoma
Cortisol secreting (basophil) adenoma
Craniopharyngioma
Meningioma
Aneurysm of the carotid artery
Secondary neoplasm
Rare infiltrations and deposits (e.g. gumma, sarcoidosis)

What problems?

Pituitary tumours (usually chromophobe) are quite commonly found routinely at postmortem but when such a tumour is found during life it must always be investigated and followed-up. Follow-up can be difficult when people have no symptoms and endocrine change, as already stated, is often insidious. However the possibility of future visual loss must always be borne in mind.

Clinical features

A slowly growing tumour may present as follows.

(1) Headache

(2) Visual deficit particularly bitemporal field encroachment

(3) Endocrine change

(4) Asymptomatic

In addition the following syndromes occur:

(1) Diabetes insipidus with upward damage to the hypothalamus or pituitary,

(2) Hypothalamic presentations (sleep disturbance, appetite disturbance etc),

(3) Pituitary apoplexy – a sudden presentation of headache, cranial nerve paresis and sometimes coma due usually to haemorrhage into a large tumour.

Assessment and investigations

(1) X-ray of the pituitary fossa usually with tomography is essential where a pituitary tumour is suspected.

(2) CAT scans can now demonstrate quite small suprasellar extensions (particularly with enhancement techniques).

(3) Visual field assessment by perimetry or central field is essential in the investigation of a pituitary tumour.

(4) Full endocrinological assessment should be made, as previously detailed.

Management

It is absolutely essential that pituitary tumours are not lost to follow-up. The following should be regularly checked at frequencies determined by individual factors:

(1) visual fields,

(2)   pituitary fossa X-rays,

(3)   CAT scans,

(4)   endocrine status.

8
DISORDERS OF THE ADRENAL GLAND

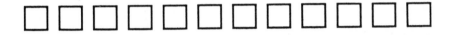

THE ADRENAL GLANDS

The adrenal glands are situated at the upper poles of the kidneys. They each comprise two distinctive histological layers – the outer cortex and the inner medulla. The cortex is further divided into three layers:

(1)　the zona glomerulosa,
(2)　the zona fasciculata,
(3)　the zona reticularis.

The embryological structure and functions of the cortex and medulla are entirely separate. They are really two distinct glands. The cortex is of mesodermal origin, secretes corticosteroids and is predominantly under the humoral control of the hypothalamus and the pituitary gland in the case of glucocorticoid secretion, and controlled via the juxtaglomerular apparatus in the case of mineralocorticoid secretion. The medulla functions as part of the autonomic nervous system and deals with the storage and secretion of adrenaline and noradrenaline. As with any other endocrine organ, disease of the adrenal is characterized by either hypofunction or hyperfunction of any of the various components of the gland.

Hormones secreted by the cortex

These are corticosteroids and all have a basic structure derived from cholesterol:

(1) Cortisol
(2) Corticosterone $\Big\}$ – the glucocorticoids
(3) Aldosterone – the mineralocorticoids
(4) Androgens – adrenal androgens include
    (a) androstenedione and
    (b) dehydroepiandrosterone (DHA)

The actions of cortisol are shown in Table 19.

Table 19 Actions of cortisol

Metabolic
Gluconeogenetic
Protein catabolic
Diabetogenic
Fat distribution altered

The inflammatory response
Most aspects inhibited

The Immune system
Humoral and cell mediated aspects both inhibited

Electrolyte balance
Sodium retaining and allows free water clearance

Mediates the body's response to 'stress'

THE FUNCTION OF THE ADRENAL GLAND

The adrenals are essential for life. The glucocorticoids, mainly through their effect on arteriolar tone and glomerular filtration rate, serve in maintaining blood pressure, but have many other actions in relation to intermediary metabolism and inflammation and wound healing (*see* Table 19).

170

The control of glucocorticoid secretion is by the action of ACTH released from the pituitary which in turn is under control from the hypothalamus. This control is mediated partly via the negative feedback mechanism already discussed for other endocrine organs. Cortisol levels also rise in reaction to stress. Levels throughout a 24 h period follow a circadian rhythm. Cortisol levels tend to be high on waking and low on retiring.

The mineralocorticoids, mainly in the form of aldosterone, control the sodium balance in the body and therefore exert an influence on the blood pressure and fluid volume by affecting the bloodflow through the juxtaglomerular apparatus. Increased levels of circulating aldosterone retain sodium, increase plasma volume and raise the blood pressure. Decreased levels of circulating aldosterone have the opposite effect. The juxtaglomerular apparatus controls aldosterone by the release of renin which in turn causes a substance called angiotensinogen, present in the plasma, to be changed to angiotensin through a converting enzyme present in the blood and the lung. This in turn exerts effects on the zona glomerulosa by releasing aldosterone.

HYPOFUNCTION OF THE ADRENAL CORTEX

This may be *primary,* as in Addison's disease or primary adrenocortical deficiency, or *secondary,* due to ACTH deficiency (*see* Chapter 7).

HYPERFUNCTION OF THE ADRENAL CORTEX

This may be due to:

(1) Cortisol excess as in Cushing's syndrome,

(2) Mineralocorticoid excess as in Conn's syndrome,

(3) Androgen excess as in virilizing syndromes,

(4) Congenital enzyme defects as in congenital adrenal hyperplasia.

171

ADDISON'S DISEASE

This was originally described in 1855 and was due to tuberculous destruction of the gland. The commonest cause now is an auto-immune adrenalitis that may be seen as part of the multiple endocrine immune disease syndrome. Other causes are:

(1)   fulminating infection (meningococcal septicaemia),
(2)   metastases,
(3)   sarcoid,
(4)   iatrogenic.

The incidence is somewhere between one in 25 000 and one in 100 000 therefore a large group practice may expect to see one case in a lifetime.

Outcome

Once diagnosed the condition is easily treatable. Replacement therapy is for life. It is of interesting historical note that John F. Kennedy was a sufferer and so probably also was Napoleon Bonaparte.

Clinical features

These are insidious and include some or all of the following:

(1)   weight loss,
(2)   fatigue,
(3)   vague gastrointestinal upset,
(4)   depression,
(5)   postural hypotension,
(6)   loss of libido,
(7)   amenorrhea,
(8)   vitiligo,
(9)   loss of body hair,

(10)   excess pigmentation along pressure areas, buccal mucosa, hand creases and light exposed areas – the excess pigmentation is associated with high circulating levels of ACTH,
(11)   electrolyte disturbances,
(12)   a low plasma sodium,
(13)   a high plasma potassium and a raised urea.

Aldosterone secretion may be preserved in the auto-immune form of disease so that electrolyte disturbances may not be a feature, and this is also seen in hypoadrenalism secondary to pituitary dysfunction.

Diagnosis

Clinical

As the disease is so uncommon and many of the features are common in other presentations of disease in a general practice clinic, the diagnosis is very likely to be missed. A point worth remembering is that a history of fatigue which increases during the day is more likely to have an organic basis. The corollary – fatigue which improves during the day – is more likely to have a functional basis.

The laboratory diagnosis

This is made by demonstrating a low level of circulating plasma cortisol, and lack of response of plasma cortisol to an injection of synthetic tetracosactrin (synacthen), an ACTH analogue.

The procedure

10 ml of heparinized blood is taken between 8.00 a.m. and 10.00 a.m. and then an injection of synacthen 250 μg i.v. is given. Plasma cortisol should rise to at least 520 nmol/l.

If the basal plasma cortisol level is less than 175 nmol/l adrenal hypofunction can be diagnosed, but many cases of Addison's disease will have a normal basal cortisol level. Blood for ACTH levels, a full blood count, autoantibodies, urea and electrotypes may also be taken at the same time. A low ACTH implies secondary adrenal hypofunction and should be investigated by an endocrinologist who will look for pituitary causes.

Remember

Adrenal insufficiency can occur in conjunction with other conditions such as thyroid disease and pernicious anaemia.

Treatment

Lifelong replacement therapy is required. The typical regime is hydrocortisone 20 mg taken in the morning and 10 mg at night. This balance is to mimic the circadian rhythm. Mineralocorticoid replacement in the form of fludrocortisone 0.1–0.2 mg daily is usually necessary in addition. Regular check-up at outpatients and by the GP is mandatory.

Educating the Patient

Make him aware of the need for lifelong treatment. Patients can carry Medicalert cards or bracelets but a special steroid card with the full dose details is better. Hospital and GP notes should be specially marked. Both patient and GP should be aware of the existence of adrenal crisis and the need for extra steroids (usually double the dose for the duration of the illness) during intercurrent infection and, if necessary, for hospital admission. Vomiting patients may need their steroid parenterally.

SUMMARY OF ADRENAL HYPOFUNCTION

(1)   It is rare.

(2)   Suspect if hyperpigmentation occurs in association with other features described.

Other causes of hyperpigmentation

These are:

(1)   ethnic,
(2)   liver disease,
(3)   carcinomatosis,
(4)   Cushing's syndrome and
(5)   pregnancy.

HYPERFUNCTION OF THE ADRENAL CORTEX: CUSHING'S SYNDROME

Cushing's syndrome arises from an excess of circulating plasma glucocorticoid. It may be primary or secondary.

Primary causes are as follows:

(1)   Adrenal adenoma

(2)   Adrenal carcinoma

Secondary causes are as follows:

(1)   Increased ACTH from pituitary = Cushing's disease (*see* Chapter 7);

(2)   Ectopic ACTH production from various tumours, the commonest being an oat cell carcinoma of the bronchus;

(3)   Iatrogenic. This is the commonest cause for Cushing's syndrome. In adrenal causes and when exogenous steroids are given ACTH is low. In pituitary hyperfunction circulating ACTH is high. When a tumour ectopically secreting ACTH is present levels are very high.

Incidence

This is not known, although the pituitary dependent form accounts for 80% of all causes of Cushing's syndrome.

Clinical features

These are as follows:

(1)   Hirsutism
(2)   Truncal obesity
(3)   Proximal myopathy
(4)   Purple striae on abdomen
(5)   Buffalo hump
(6)   Acne
(7)   Collapsing vertebrae
(8)   Menstrual disturbances
(9)   Loss of libido
(10) Diabetes
(11) Hypertension

The striae should be differentiated from those seen in pregnancy and large adolescent girls.

Hyperpigmentation may also be present due to the high ACTH.

Visual field defects may be present due to an expanding pituitary tumour, but this is very rare unless the patient has already had a bilateral adrenalectomy.

Establishing the diagnosis

Clinical

This may well be picked up in general practice. A patient record review can be useful if the disease is suspected. Check for recent or long term weight gain, blood pressure readings, routine urinalysis. Note the presence or absence of hirsuties. The most important thing is to view the appearance of the whole body, presenting with thin arms and legs and a rounded trunk and face.

Biochemical diagnosis – Screening

This is done by the overnight dexamethasone test and can easily be performed in general practice. The object is to demonstrate high levels of circulating cortisol and loss of the circadian rhythm. Dexamethasone suppresses ACTH and hence cortisol release in normal subjects but does not interfere with the laboratory measurement of endogenous cortisol. In Cushing's disease morning cortisol levels are not suppressed after the dose of dexamethasone.

Procedure

Prescribe 2 mg of oral dexamethasone to be taken at 10.00 p.m. At 8.00 a.m. the following day take 10 ml of heparinized blood for plasma cortisol. If the plasma cortisol is greater than 175 mmol/l then referral to an endocrinologist is mandatory to determine whether the cause is primary or secondary. Investigations will include pituitary function and screening for tumours. In spite of highly sophisticated investigations it is still often difficult to detect an underlying neoplasm (see Chapter 7).

Treatment of Cushing's syndrome

This depends on the cause. The aim is to remove the source(s) of excess cortisol and effect a return to physiological levels of secretion. Treatment of Cushing's syndrome is not ideal.

Adrenal tumours

These are resected where possible.

Ectopic ACTH secreting tumours

Surgery followed by radiotherapy is the present mode of therapy.

These tumours have a high morbidity and rapid progression. Drugs such as adrenal blocking agents, metyrapone and amino-glutethimide may be useful. The adrenal cell toxic agent o.p. DDD can be useful, but is very toxic.

Cushing's disease caused by ACTH secreting pituitary tumour

See Chapter 7 for details of this condition.

HYPERALDOSTERONISM

This is *Conn's syndrome*, resulting from an excess of circulating mineralocorticoids. This is thought to be due to hyperfunction of the zona glomerulosa in association with an aldosterone secreting adenoma, microadenomata or hyperplasia.

Incidence

The incidence has been found in some series to be as high as 1% of the hypertensive population and is potentially therefore of considerable clinical significance to both hospital and general practitioner. However, such an incidence is not the experience of most British endocrinologists.

Clinical features

These include weakness or paralysis, polyuria, polydipsia, hypertension and metabolic alkalosis. Oedema does not generally occur. The features are caused in general by either sodium retention or hypokalaemia.

Differential diagnosis includes:

(1)   renal disease,

(2)   tetany,

(3)   myasthenia gravis,

(4)   all forms of secondary hyperaldosteronism such as malignant
       hypertension, liver disease, cardiac failure etc.

Conn's syndrome may be masked or mimicked by the use of
diuretics or substances such as biogastrone which cause hypokalaemia. Old blood and therefore inaccurate laboratory results
will also confuse diagnosis. If the diagnosis is suspected, fresh
plasma from a non-occluded vessel will help to minimize errors. If
there is doubt about interference by drugs, the drugs can be stopped and urine potassium levels measured after 10 days. A 24 h
urinary potassium excretion of greater than 50 mmol in the presence of a low serum potassium concentration is very suggestive of
hyperaldosteronism (not necessarily primary).

Specialist tests

These include plasma renin and plasma aldosterone measurement.

In primary aldosteronism the aldosterone will be high and the
renin will be low. A high plasma renin occurs in secondary aldosteronism such as malignant hypertension and renal artery stenosis.
Sodium loading and depletion tests are also helpful as are serum
renin measurements in the erect and supine positions. In Conn's
syndrome these manoeuvres do not alter what is usually autonomous oversecretion of aldosterone with renin suppression.

Localization

Once primary aldosteronism has been established the following
may be helpful in localization : i.v.u., CAT scan, adrenal angio-
gram, adrenal scan with labelled cholesterol, selective adrenal vein
sampling.

Treatment

(1) Removal of cause if surgically possible.

Remember that glucocorticoid and mineralocorticoid cover will be required.

(2) The use of an aldosterone antagonist such as spironolactone which may have to be given in large quantities up to 400 mg/day.

Remember : spironolactone can cause painful and cosmetically unacceptable gynaecomastia.

HYPERFUNCTION AND ABNORMALITIES OF ADRENAL ANDROGENS

Brief mention of these may be made here. Benign *adenomas* may be virilizing. Carcinomas tend to have mixed glucocorticoid and androgenic effects. If adenoma or carcinoma is suspected, investigation should be made by an endocrinologist.

CONGENITAL ADRENAL HYPERPLASIA

This occurs consequent to an inborn error of metabolism, resulting in a total or partial deficiency of one of several enzymes involved in the biosynthesis of steroids. The commonest type is 21-hydroxylase block. This is an inherited autosomal recessive condition resulting in a failure to convert 17-OH progesterone to 11-deoxycortisol and thence cortisol. There is a state of relative lack of cortisol (which can lead to adrenal collapse) and sometimes also aldosterone. This in turn leads to high ACTH levels which stimulate mass production of adrenal androgens. The condition causes masculinization of the female neonate or the 'infant Hercules' appearance of male children. Milder forms exist which can present as hirsutism in a child or young woman. In the established condition, both male and female tend to be of short stature due to premature closure of the epiphyses. The best single investigation is the serum 17-OH progesterone level, which is raised in affected cases. Prednisolone is the lifelong treatment. This suppresses the high ACTH levels to normal. 11-Hydroxylase deficiency causes androgenization but with salt retention. Other rarer forms will not be dealt with.

DISORDERS OF THE ADRENAL MEDULLA

The adrenal medulla comprises cords of chromatin cells. It is really part of the autonomic nervous system with a nerve supply equivalent to the postganglionic sympathetic nerve fibre. The medulla stores, synthesizes and secretes catecholamines in the form of adrenaline and noradrenaline. Their release is under central nervous control and occurs in response to:

(1) hypoglycaemia,
(2) hypotension,
(3) stress.

Pheochromocytomas

These are rare tumours of chromatin tissue which secrete an excess of catecholamines. They are uncommon but do account for a small proportion of cases of hypertension. The incidence is somewhat less than one in 10 000. They may be multiple, present in the gland itself or located ectopically anywhere along the sympathetic nerve chain. About 10% of pheochromocytomas are malignant, and there may be a family history with autosomal dominant inheritance.

Clinical features

These reflect excess α- and β-adrenoreceptor stimulation and effects vary as whether noradrenaline (α-agonist) or adrenaline (α- and β-agonist) is predominantly secreted (Table 20).

181

Table 20   α-Effects and β-effects of adrenaline

α-Effects	β-Effects
Hypertension (intermittent or sustained)	Flushing
	Palpitations
Anxiety	Tachydysrhythmias
Angina	Sweating
Pallor	Fever
	Hyperglycaemia

Occasionally other neuroectodermal abnormalities are found, such as neurofibromata and café-au-lait spots.

The diagnosis is made by demonstrating a high level of circulating catecholamine metabolites in the urine. The commonest method is by measuring vanilylmandelic acid (VMA) in a 24 h specimen in conjunction with the serum creatinine. Concomitant hypotensive therapy with methyldopa or a diet high in bananas can interfere with this test. Other tests are then needed to localize the tumour. These are best carried out in specialist clinics and have been previously referred to.

Management

This involves surgical removal if possible. Before surgery α- and β-blocking drugs are given and the management both before and after surgery is not simple.

The diagnosis, treatment and follow-up of pheochromocytoma is complex and should be controlled by specialist clinics. There is a considerable morbidity attached to the condition.

SUMMARY

Diseases of the adrenal gland are rare but have an undeserved reputation for 'difficulty'. They can usually be recognized and initially investigated by the GP. Once hypo- or hyperfunction has been detected, referral to a specialist clinic is mandatory in most cases.

Follow-up after treatment and monitoring replacement therapy can be done jointly.

Patient education is essential.

Index

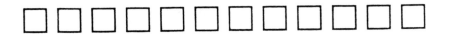

185